Stingless Bees' Impact on Human Health & Uses in Traditional Remedies

Abu Hassan Jalil

To order additional copies of this book, contact:
Xlibris
844-714-8691
www.Xlibris.com
Orders@Xlibris.com

ISBN:	Softcover	978-1-6698-7970-1
	Hardcover	978-1-6698-7969-5
	EBook	978-1-6698-7971-8

Print information available on the last page

Rev. date: 06/07/2023

SYNOPSIS

A study on how Stingless Bee culturing and the impact of its products on human socio-economic, health and well-being development. From its ancient initiation to the evolution of the current methods and techniques, it includes traditional practices across many ethnic beliefs and lifestyles. For example, Stingless bee honey is a popular traditional medicine that traditional practitioners use to treat various disorders, particularly respiratory and gastrointestinal disorders.

A section on taste profiles explores new or improved tastes with herbal and spice infusions and mixes for more palatable healthy drinks and commercially viable culinary products. It also looks at Vinaigrettes, salad dressing and marinades.

This book makes comparisons of different vegetation exudates and nectar of different crop blossoms. It explains how the resulting products like honey, propolis and pollen derived from meliponiculture are used and how they impact human health.

ABSTRACT

This presentation is representative of Stingless Bee Derivatives & By-Products and their impact on human health. Emphasis is on Indo-Malayan Stingless Bees, their traditional uses in ASEAN countries, and the influence of Middle Eastern traditions, practices and Islamic concepts.

The ASEAN traditions are from indigenous peoples and knowledge from ancient Indian Ayurvedic, Traditional Chinese Medical (TCM) practices assimilated into the total Asian culture. Derivative products range from Honey - Wound Treatment & Body care; Wax – Candles, Polishes and Protective Coats; Propolis – Termite Repellents, Stains, Poultices and Wood & Leather Preservatives; Pollen & Propolis – Poultry Feed. Other products in the form of consumables are: Honey – Raw, Maceration & Infusions, Vinaigrettes & Salad Dressing & Marinades; Propolis – Nutraceuticals, Hydrosols Pharmaceuticals & Sterilized Capsules in oral consumption for well-being and health supplement; Pollen – Raw or sterilized & encapsulated, Power Muesli Bars & Healthy Culinary Desserts; Larvae – Raw or processed (grilled)

Traditional Folk Remedies encompasses herbal honey remedies handed down from generations of indigenous people guided by ancient knowledge, including alternative medical practice from traditional medicine in China. Herbal-based but can sometimes include minerals. Arabic and Islamic Religious concepts and philosophies. Not overlooking Quranic verses and Hadiths [i.e., sayings and deeds of the Prophet (PBUH)]. Honey Alchemy (from the times of the Pharaohs when Honey was found in the tombs of the Pyramids) to develop the elixir of life - so pure it promises youth, beauty and longevity. These quests forge the indigenous knowledge and information condensed in this presentation.

The regional cultures from the countries explored are Malaysia, Thailand, Indonesia, Philippines and some Middle Eastern and Islamic communities in the Indo-Malayan Ecozone. The products examined are derived from: Orchards and plantations practising Meliponiculture: Wild SB Honey and Honeybees; Farmed Monoculture Nectar; Maceration & Infusion of domestic Honey; and other Product derivatives & concoctions.

Keywords: Raw Honey, Maceration, Infusion, Dominant nectar, Derivative products, ASEAN traditions, Middle East & Islamic, Ayurveda & TCM.

CONTENTS

PREFACE

Inspiration from the Holy Scriptures

As mentioned in Al-Quran, Surah An-Nahl verses 68 to 69 ('Ali, 1999), Your Lord inspired the bee, saying: "Set up hives in the mountains and the trees and in the trellises (structures) that people put up. Then suck the juice of every kind of fruit and keep treading the ways of your Lord which have been made easy." There comes forth from their bellies a drink varied in colours, wherein there is **healing for men.** Verily there is a sign in this for those who reflect".

A decade of travelling in the ASEAN region and Australia abounded me with many uses of honey and the traditional uses practised as folk hone-remedies. Many of the practices may be unfounded; however, in most instances, albeit some weird myths, I have gathered reference articles in journals of human health and ancient practices, like the Indian Ayurvedic principles and Traditional Chines Medicine (TCM) and Taoist Alchemy. In some Muslim communities, there is adherence to Islamic concepts and philosophy.

After practising Meliponiculture for almost a dozen years, we have always put Beescape as the top priority in all considerations regarding farm management for Meliponaries incorporated in Orchards or plantations. From that, we see some relation and influence Beescape has on honey production. The type of crops and season, too, had a direct relation to the moisture content of the resultant harvested honey. We had difficulty quantifying the relation because the bees are polylectic in that they forage whichever source was available then.

However, we can predict an estimated volume of regularly scheduled harvesting in monoculture farms or forests with a dominant vegetation type. In such instances, we can ascertain the peculiar benefits that we may get from the types of honey. Another instance is where the bee is affixed to a certain type of vegetation and is even dependent on such vegetation. A good example is the species that depend on Dipterocarp resin; in that way, we will be sure that the honey will have resinous micro propolis. This affinity will influence the taste, aroma and, to a certain extent, the colour.

Introduction

Meliponiculture has its benefits and hurdles as well. The benefits naturally come in health and wealth if done patiently and diligently. To reap the benefits, one must also withstand and overcome extremes in seasonal climate plus occasional pest and predator infestation. Dedication and full concentration of efforts in proper Meliponary management is crucial. Control of a buffer perimeter and wind barrier to keep potential use of pesticides in the surrounding neighbouring area. The appropriate bee forage needs, and grounds upkeep require the right amount of labour reciprocated with the appropriate density of hives within the farm area.

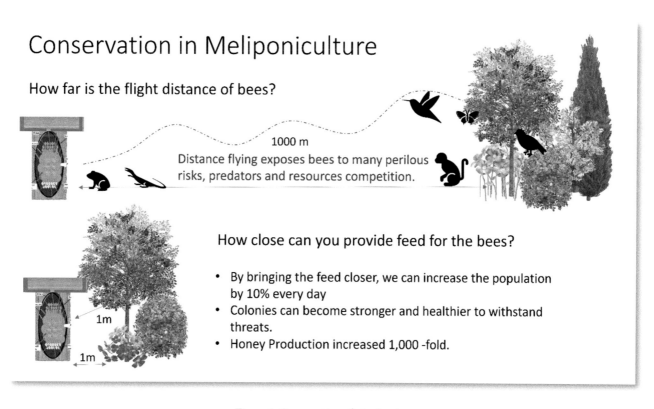

Figure 1 Conservation of stingless bees

Conservation of stingless bees must be continuous in meliponary management. Bee scientists, entomologists and researchers frequently scrutinize the bees' flight range and forage distances. This data need not be crucial information for a beekeeper. The keeper's more important concern should be how close they can provide foraging sources. The further the distance the bee travels, the greater the dangers they face. Besides predators and pests, they face extreme weather changes like a sudden downpour of strong gales that can divert their return path or the scent trail of their forage destination. These conditions also reduce the productivity of the whole colony.

Traditional Folk Remedies

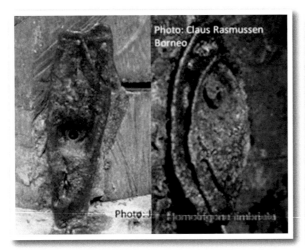

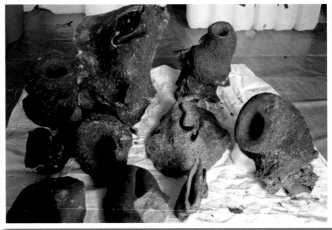

Figure 3 Ovoid shape (Introitus) nest entrance cerumen

Figure 2 Geniotrigona thoracica and G. lacteifasciata nest entrance funnels

Ovoid shape (Introitus) nest entrance cerumen and ovaloid gyne cells are proposed as gynaecological ailment remedies for women, such as increasing breast milk production, relieving menstrual cramps, and increasing sex drive.

Geniotrigona thoracica and *G. lacteifasciata* nest entrance funnels pulverized and glycol extracted to treat piles.

Many of these herbal honey remedies were handed down from generations of indigenous people guided by ancient knowledge, e.g.:

- Indian Ayurvedic medicinal practices – Honey is used for urinary tract disorders, bronchial asthma, coughs, diarrhoea, nausea, and vomiting.
- Traditional Chinese medicine (TCM) is an alternative medical practice drawn from traditional medicine in China. Herbal-based but can sometimes include minerals.
- Arabic and Islamic Religious concepts and philosophies. Quranic verses and Hadiths [sayings and deeds of the Prophet (pbuh)]
- Honey Alchemy (from the times of the Pharaohs when Honey was found in the tombs of the Pyramids) to develop the elixir of life – so pure it promises youth, beauty and longevity.

*All medicinal properties proposed herein are speculative and are based on traditional beliefs and hearsay unless otherwise referenced in published journal articles[1].

The Good, The Myth & The Weird

Honey bee broods (larvae and pupae) are nontoxic and have a very rich nutritional value, presenting a high content of protein and fat similar to beef, but richer in minerals and most vitamins

In addition, the bee brood was a good source of essential amino acids, with methionine being the first limiting. While the bee brood contained none of the fat-soluble vitamins (vitamins A, D, and E), it was a good source of most B vitamins and vitamin C and choline.

Holding the brood is the honeycomb, rich in healthy carbohydrates and antioxidants, which can boost the immune system. The beeswax in honeycomb also contains long-chain fatty acids, which are good for the heart and lowering bad cholesterol levels. In addition, beeswax contains natural alcohols with hepatoprotective qualities.

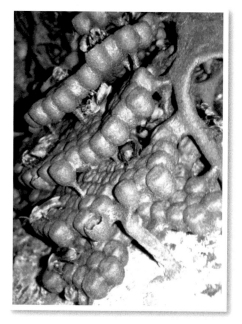

Figure 4 Stingless bee Pre pupa comb brood

In Kampuchea, a Honeycomb bee brood is grilled for human consumption. In Sabah, some indigenous tribes eat *H. itama* and *G. thoracica* brood raw.

North Borneo Kadazan, Dusun & Murut consume bee larvae for aphrodisiac revitalization.

1   Ismail, N. F. ., Zulkifli, M. F., & Wan Ismail, W. I. (2022). Therapeutic Potentials of Bee Products for Treatment of COVID-19. IIUM Medical Journal Malaysia, 21(1). https://doi.org/10.31436/imjm.v21i1.1893

CHAPTER 2

Uses of Stingless Bee Products

- Honey Wound Treatment, Body care
- Wax – Candles, Polishes and Protective Coats
- Propolis – Termite Repellents, Stains, Poultices and Wood & Leather Preservatives
- Pollen & Propolis – Poultry Feed
- Pollination services

Consumables

- Honey – Raw, Maceration & Infusions, Pickles (Jeruk, Acar)
- Propolis – Nutraceuticals, Hydrosols Pharmaceuticals & Capsules.
- Pollen – Raw, Power Muesli Bars & Healthy Culinary Desserts & Sauces
- Larvae – Raw or processed
- Alcoholic Wines & Liqueurs
- Vinaigrettes & Salad Dressing & Marinades

Types of Products

The homey types scrutinized herein are:

- Meliponiculture and Apiculture
- Wild SB Honey and Honeybees
- Farmed Monoculture Nectar
- Maceration & Infusion
- Product derivatives & concoctions

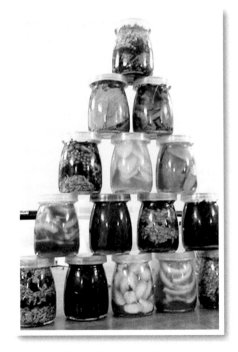

Figure 5 Spice & Herbal Maceration & Honey Infusion

Spice & Herbal Maceration & Honey Infusion

- Black cumin (Habatus sauda) *Nigella sativa*
- Cinnamon/Pepper/Fenugreek/Cloves & Five spice – Clove, Star Anise, Fennel, Cumin, Caraway
- Ginger/ Turmeric/ Garlic/ Lemon/ Nutmeg/
- Sea-Cucumber/Seagarapes/ Peperomia/ Salam leaves
- Tongkat Ali (*Eurycoma longifolia*)

Raw Honey Taste profile[2]

Ayurveda identifies 6 Tastes by which all foods can be categorized: Sweet, Sour, Salty, Bitter, Pungent, and Astringent.

- On average, the Meliponine raw honey is sweet and sour. *Tetragonula* honey is sweeter than sour with some of them, like *T. fuscobalteata* being sweet with a tinge of sourness, while *T. melanocephala* is more sour than sweet.
- This taste is the same with the underground types like *Tetragonilla collina* and *T. atripes,* i.e., more sour than sweet.
- *Lophotrigona canifrons,* on the other end, is astringent, and others in between are rather tart to sour, and we rarely get the domesticated version of L. canifrons because of its ferocity.
- Other sour ones, like *Homotrigona fimbriata, Tetrigona apicalis,* or *Tetrigona binghami, can sometimes be so astringent tha*t they can be non-palatable in raw form.
- *Geniotrigona thoracica* has a savoury flavour with a tinge of tart after-taste. *Heterotrigona itama* is equally savoury but with a bitter after-taste, especially from wild *Acacia* sp. forest. *Lepidotrigona sp.* honey has a sweet and sour taste.

With these profiles, one may explore new or improved tastes with herbal infusions and mixes for more platable healthy drinks and commercially viable culinary products.

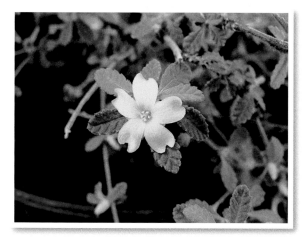

Figure 6 Turnera diffusa var. aphrodisiaca, Turneraceae, Damiana, flower.

Turnera Honey Liqueur

While on the topic of libido and aphrodisiacs the *Turnera diffusa* var. *aphrodisiaca,* Turneraceae, Damiana, flower. The name speaks for itself.

- *Turnera ulmifolia* (Yellow Alder) in South America and the West Indies traditional medicine, a tea made from the leaves of this species is used to treat gastrointestinal problems (constipation, diarrhoea), colds and flu, vascular diseases (heart palpitations), menstrual cramps, and dermatological issues.

---

2   http://www.eattasteheal.com/ETH_6tastes.htm

- *Turnera subulata* blooms usually at 08.00 am and can last up to 5 years under proper maintenance schedules.

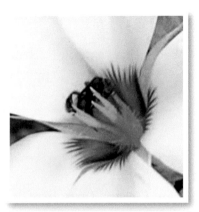

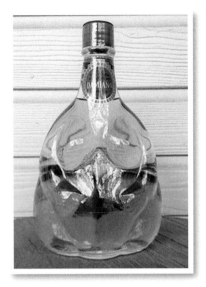

- Souza, C.N., et al., 20116 *Turnera subulata Anti-Inflammatory Properties in Lipopolysaccharide-Stimulated RAW 264.7 Macrophages JOURNAL OF MEDICINAL FOOD J Med Food 19 (10) 2016, 922–930 DOI: 10.1089/jmf.2016.0047*

A bottle of Damiana liqueur: is an alcoholic drink composed of spirits (often rectified spirits) and additional flavourings such as honey, fruits, herbs, and spices [3].

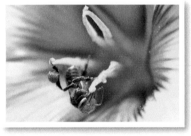

Figure 8 A bottle of Damiana liqueur

Figure 7 Turnera subulata

Sauces, Cider and Wines

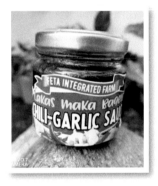

Philippines Stingless bee pollen is one of the ingredients in a Chilly-garlic sauce... Local name = Lakas Makabagets in Bicol.

A pollen-derivative beverage is Farm Tomato mush distilled and fermented with Meliponine derived pollen. This beverage is a cottage industry product as a fruit wine in Iloilo, Panay.

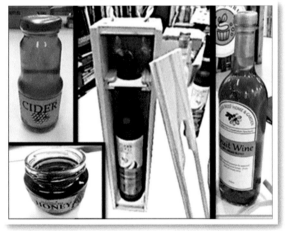

Figure 9 Lakas Makabagets

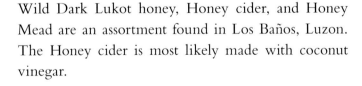

Wild Dark Lukot honey, Honey cider, and Honey Mead are an assortment found in Los Baños, Luzon. The Honey cider is most likely made with coconut vinegar.

Folk Remedies Using Herbal and Spices Honey Infusion

- Garlic, ginger and lemon honey. This supplement helps with cholesterol and congestive heart problems.
- Garlic honey. It is good for prolonged fever problems and a body with less disease resistance.
- Turmeric Honey great for the skin, good for your digestive systems, are rich in antioxidants, healing wounds & burns

---

3   https://en.wikipedia.org/wiki/Turnera_diffusa#/media/File:DamianaLiqueur.jpg.

- Ginger honey promotes the secretion of bile and intestinal flora, which helps dissolve fat. Help soothe the side effects of chemotherapy, like nausea and vomiting.
- Ginger Lemon Honey reduces kidney damage. Reduce the risk and effects of diabetes. Increased brain health. Improved skin appearance.
- Tongkat Ali sweet honey is in demand for erectile dysfunction ailments.

Traditional herbal concoctions for female health

Labisia pumila (Kacip Fatimah) + Honey Beverage

A.k.a. Selusuh Fatimah

Selusuh is used as an effort to facilitate women in giving birth.

Benefits are: To Slow Down Aging. Anti-Oxidative. Herbal Menopause Relief... Nourish the Skin... Keep Skin Hydration... Rejuvenating Action.

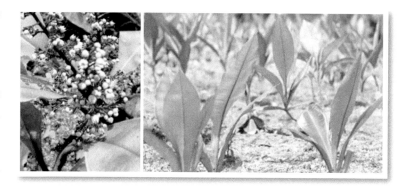

Figure 12 Labisia pumila (Kacip Fatimah)

Kacip Fatimah has been traditionally used by Malay women for many generations in childbirth to induce and eases delivery, as a post-partum medication to help the birth channel, to regain body strength, regulate the menstrual cycle and avoid pain and alleviate menopausal symptoms[4].

Commercially canned drinks are available as flavoured drinks with Kacip Fatimah and Honey Dates.

References

- Manda, V. K., et al. *Evaluation of Drug Interaction Potential of Labisia pumila (Kacip Fatimah) and Its Constituents* Frontiers in Pharmacology August 2014 | Volume5 | Article 178 | **1** doi: 10.3389/fphar.2014.00178
- Zakaria, AA et al., 2021, *A Review on Therapeutic Effects of Labisia pumila on Female Reproductive Diseases* Hindawi BioMed Research International Volume 2021, Article ID 9928199, 9 pages <u>https://doi.org/10.1155/2021/9928199</u>

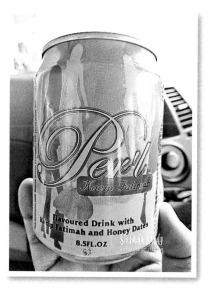

Figure 11 Kacip Fatimah and Honey Dates.

---

4   Web ref: http://www.myhealth.gov.my/en/kacip-fatimah-2/
https://upm.edu.my/news/efficacy_of_kacip_fatimah_is_not_a_myth_says_award_winning_upm_researcher-24889

Quercus infectoria (Manjakani or Majuphal) & Honey Mix

In Ayurveda, it has been successfully used for controlling loose motions[5], women's reproductive problems and vaginal discharge. A decoction from Majuphal treats skin problems, sore throat and stomatitis.

Mayaphala (Majuphal) is an Ayurvedic herb used to treat wounds, control bleeding, piles, oral diseases, diarrhoea, dysmenorrhea and cases of plant poisoning.

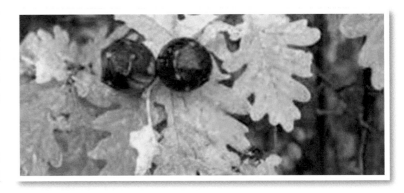

Figure 13 Quercus infectoria (Manjakani or Majuphal)

Manjakani, or its scientific name *Quercus infectoria,* is a plant or tree with other names such as Oak Tree, Oak Galls or Mecca Manjakani. For some countries like China, Arab, India, Malaysia, Brunei and Iran, Manjakani is used in herbal ingredients.

The Benefits of Manjakani for Women's Health[6]

There are many benefits, especially in terms of health, treatment of diseases and treatment of female organs.

- Maintaining The Health of Women's Intimate Organs
- Its usefulness to the female organs includes overcoming excessive fluid, killing bacteria and fungi, making it tighter, and increasing the elasticity of the vaginal muscle area.
- The Pharmacological Journal recorded that Manjakani extract contains nutrients and compounds that have anti-inflammatory, anti-diabetic, antimicrobial, and Astringent.
- According to an expert named Prof. Dr. Hembing Wijayakusuma, in addition to overcoming Leucorrhoea, reducing fluids, and improving the elasticity of female organs,
- In Aceh, Manjakani is usually used as a contraceptive tool for family planning. Although it also has the properties to heal wounds, it is sometimes processed and made to delay the pregnancy.
- One of the benefits of Manjakani fruits in terms of healing disease is to overcome Cyst disease. Mixed with some other natural ingredients, It is one of the recipes called Jamu Manjakani Aceh.

---

5   https://www.amazon.in/Majuphal-Masikkai-Quercus-Infectoria-Quality/dp/B07CBCR9YT

6   https://www.mamitacare.com/manjakani/5-benefits-of-manjakani-for-women-health/

CHAPTER 3

SB Honey Vinaigrettes, Salad Dressing

A simple recipe for vinaigrette or Salad Dressing is basically [one sour, one sweet, one herb(aromatic), one spice (flavour), and one creamy or savoury. The typical ratio for a vinaigrette is three parts (oil + herbs and spices) to one part sour honey or Stingless bee.

- A vegetable oil for your base
- A fragrant oil mix like Sesame seed oil for some flavour complexity and creaminess
- Stingless Bee honey (of a species that has naturally high acidity) Dipterocarp-dependent species can be very sour but with a little sweetness that does away with the need for vinegar
- Some aromatic herbs like Garlic or a fragrant leafy condiment like parsley or basil for oomph
- Salt and pepper plus a couple of spices from the 'five-spice' mix (Clove, Star Anise, Fennel, Cumin, Caraway or Cinnamon) to taste

Marinades:

Here is something for mutton, lambs and sheep meat. It may include Venison.

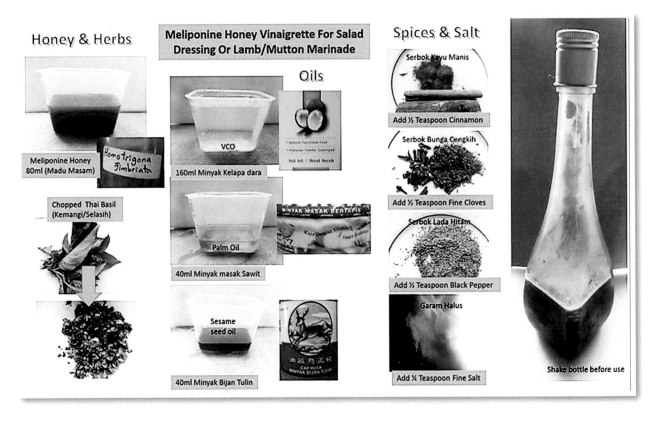

Figure 14 Meliponine Honey Vinaigrette for salad dressing or Lamb/Mutton marinades

This recipe is especially great if used with *Homotrigona fimbriata* honey. The author finds that the earthy yet sour profile goes well with Thai basil, VCO Palm oil, some sesame seed oil, cinnamon clove, and pepper.

a) *Homotrigona fimbriata* honey
b) VCO & Palm oil
c) Thai Basil
d) Sesame seed oil
e) Spices: Cinnamon, Cloves & Pepper

Muttons, lambs and sheep meat are fatty and smelly. Basil and sesame oil may counter these smells. Cloves and cinnamon bring the smells to a pleasant fragrance. The sourness and acidity of the honey will make it more savoury and flavorful.

1. This one here is for Freshwater fish or Sirloin Beef

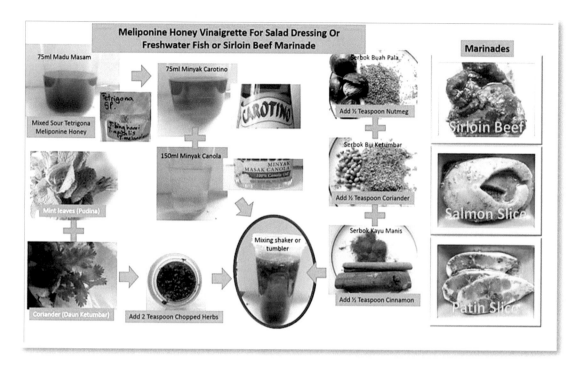

Figure 15 Meliponine Honey Vinaigrette for salad dressing or Freshwater fish and Sirloin Beef marinades

The tartness of *Tetrigona binghami, T. melanoleuca* or *T. apicalis* Honey blends well with chopped mint and coriander with base oils mix of Carotino (red palm oil) and Canola oil with spices like ground nutmeg, coriander seed and cinnamon.

2. For Ocean Fish Marinade, one may try this.

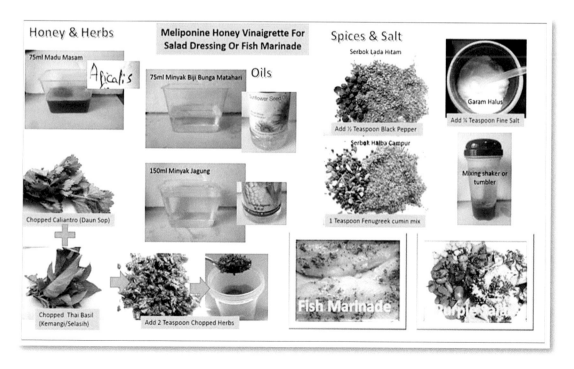

Figure 16 Meliponine Honey Vinaigrette for salad dressing or Freshwater fish and Sirloin Beef marinades

With astringent wild *T. apicalis and T. peninsularis* honey, we add cilantro and basil to Sunflower seed oil and corn oil and spice up with pepper and fenugreek. Great for a purple salad consisting of purple cabbage, red beans and beetroot.

a) *Tetrigona apicalis* or *T. peninsularis* honey
b) Sun Flower seed & Corn oil
c) Thai Basil & Cilantro (may opt for Thyme & Oregano)
d) Spices: Fenugreek & Pepper
e) Salt to taste

The fenugreek and pepper, if roasted first, are excellent for ridding of fishy smells.

3. For Beef marinade

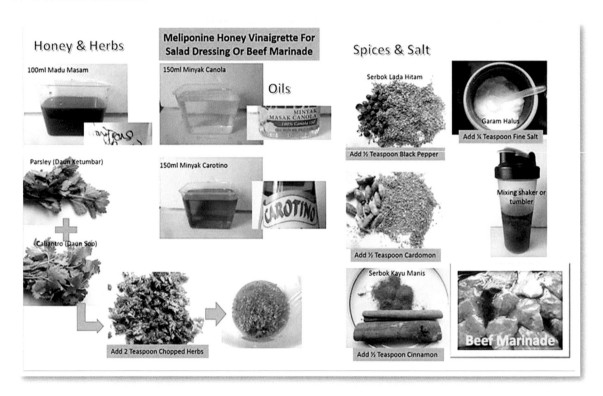

Figure 17 Meliponine Honey Vinaigrette for salad dressing or Buffalo or Beef marinades

The highly astringent Honey of Lophotrigona canifrons is good for Buffalo meat and Beef marination. Add chopped coriander and cilantro to Red Palm oil and Canola oil. Spice up with Pepper, Cardamon and Cinnamon.

a) *Lophotrigona canifrons* honey
b) Red Palm oil & Canola oil
c) Coriander & cilantro (may opt for Rosemary & Sage)
d) Spices: Cardamon, Cinnamon & Pepper
e) Salt to taste

4. Zesty Chicken Marinade

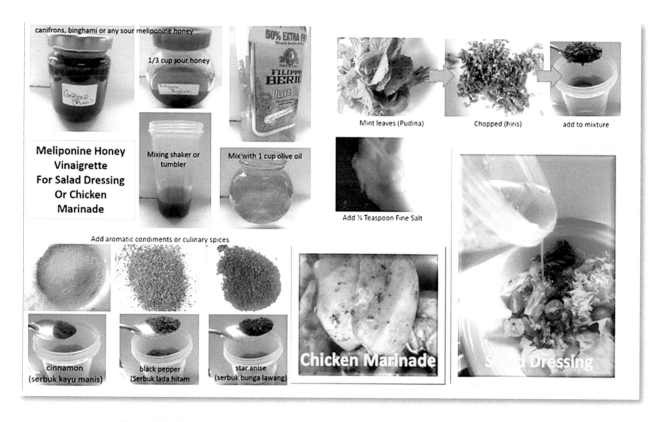

Figure 18 Meliponine Honey Vinaigrette for salad dressing or Turkey or Chicken marinades

This recipe calls for any sour honey like *T. binghami* or *L. canifrons*. Spiced up with cinnamon, star anise and pepper. The base oil is virgin olive with chopped mint leaves, which can also be basil.

a) 1/3 cup *Lophotrigona canifrons* or *Tetrigona binghami* sour honey
b) 1 cup Virgin Olive oil
c) Chopped mint or basil (may opt for thyme and Rosemary)
d) Spices: Star anise, Cinnamon & Pepper
e) Salt to taste

CHAPTER 4

Bee Pollen & Propolis Extracts - Hydrosol from the Philippines

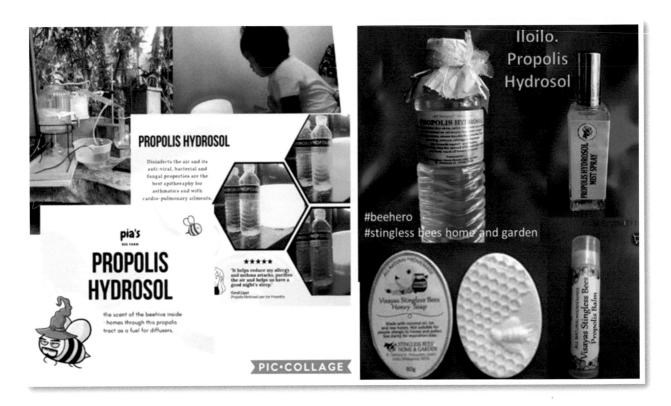

Figure 19 Propolis Hydrosol in the Philippines

Propolis Hydrosols are produced by steam distillation of meliponine propolis. It is antibacterial, antifungal and antiviral. Applied with an atomizer helps asthmatic-prone sufferers and respiratory ailments.

Propolis throat spray soothes your throat with its high content of propolis. Bee Propolis is nature's ultimate protector and is the hive's immune system. It has been used for centuries for immune support, soothing scratchy larynx, and overall health and wellness. Source: https://www.honeygreen.com/propolis-throat-spray-all-you-need-to-consider-to-prepare-the-formula/

References:

1. Hossain *et al.*, 2022 *Propolis: An update on its chemistry and pharmacological applications* Chinese Medicine (2022) 17:100 https://doi.org/10.1186/s13020-022-00651-2
2. Alanazi, S. 2022, *Antineoplastic and Antitrypanosomal Properties of Propolis from Tetragonula biroi Friese.* Molecules 2022, 27, 7463. https://doi.org/10.3390/molecules27217463
3. Desamero, M.J., et al., 2019, *Tumor-suppressing potential of stingless bee propolis in vitro and in vivo models of differentiated type gastric adenocarcinoma* **Scientific Reports** | *(2019) 9:19635* | https://doi.org/10.1038/s41598-019-55465-4

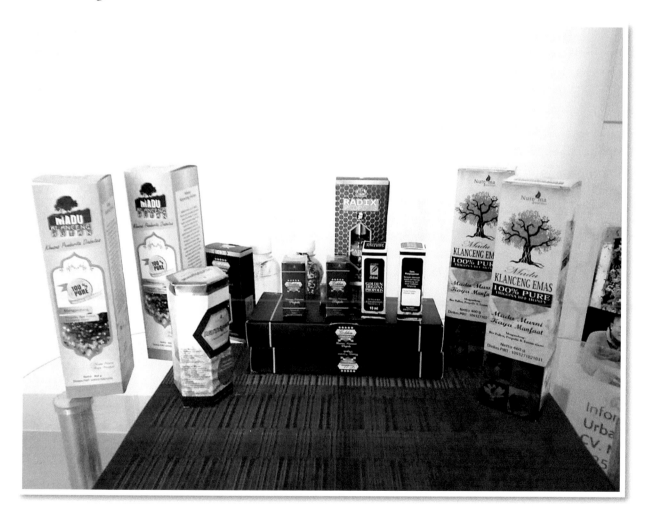

Figure 20 Propolis products in Indonesia

Meliponine propolis-based products from Java

Healing compounds in propolis[7]

Researchers have identified more than 500 (trusted source) compounds in propolis. The majority of these compounds are forms of polyphenols. Polyphenols are antioxidants that fight disease and damage in the body.

Specifically, propolis contains polyphenols called flavonoids. Flavonoids are produced in plants as a form of protection. They're commonly found in foods thought to have antioxidant properties, including fruits, green tea, vegetables, red wine

Propolis also contains other potential healing compounds, such as amino acids, vitamins A, C, and E, and minerals, such as potassium and magnesium. Other components naturally found in propolis include pollen, wax, and resin.

Propolis is thought to have antibacterial, antiviral, antifungal, antioxidant and anti-inflammatory properties. Research suggests that these may translate to the following benefits[8]:

Wounds

Propolis has a special compound called pinocembrin, a flavonoid that acts as an antifungal. These anti-inflammatory and antimicrobial properties make propolis helpful in treating wounds such as burns.

One 2019 review also notes that propolis may help stimulate collagen production in the skin, which could further support wound healing.

Cold sores and genital herpes

Ointments that contain 3% propolis, such as Herstat or Coldsore-FX, may help speed healing time and reduce symptoms in both cold sores and sores from genital herpes.

One study found that topical propolis was applied three times a day. It helped to heal cold sores faster than no treatment. The researchers found the propolis cream not only reduced the amount of herpes virus present in a person's body but also protected the body against future cold sore breakouts.

Oral Health

Another 2021 review found propolis may help treat mouth and throat infections and dental caries (cavities). Here, researchers suggest the product's antibacterial and anti-inflammatory effects could affect oral health care.

---

7   https://www.meliponinibeehoney.com/store/products/melipona-stingless-raw-propolis-extract-75-pack-of-5-sprays-2-fl-oz-60-ml

8   https://www.healthline.com/health/propolis-an-ancient-healer

Cancer

Propolis has been suggested to have a role in treating certain cancers as well. According to one 2021 study, propolis may: keep cancerous cells from multiplying, reduce the likelihood cells will become cancerous; block pathways that keep cancer cells from signalling to each other; reduce side effects of certain cancer treatments, such as chemotherapy and radiation therapy; Researchers also suggested that propolis could be a complementary therapy — but not a sole treatment — for cancer.

Chronic diseases

Research suggests that some of the anti-oxidative effects of propolis may have potential cardiovascular, neurological, and anti-diabetic benefits.

According to one 2019 review, polyphenol-rich foods and supplements like propolis may reduce the risk of high cholesterol, heart disease, and stroke.

The same review also noted that propolis might possess neuroprotective effects against multiple sclerosis (M.S.), Parkinson's disease, and dementia. Still, as with other purported benefits of propolis, more research is needed to confirm where such supplements may help prevent neurological disorders.

Additionally, a 2022 review suggests that propolis may have implications in preventing and treating type 2 diabetes. It's thought that its flavonoids could potentially help control insulin release.

However, it's unclear whether propolis alone could offer any of the above benefits, and if so, in what doses. Source: https://www.healthline.com/health/propolis-an-ancient-healer#research

References:

- Agussalim, 2021, The physicochemical composition of Honey from Indonesian stingless bee (Tetragonula laeviceps) BIODIVERSITAS Volume 22, Number 8, August 2021 Pages: 3257-3263 DOI: 10.13057/biodiv/d220820
- Harianja, A.H., et al., 2023, *Potential of Beekeeping to Support the Livelihood, Economy, Society, and Environment of Indonesia.* Forests 2023, 14, 321. https://doi.org/10.3390/f14020321
- Gratzer, K., 2019, *Challenges for Beekeeping in Indonesia with Autochthonous and Introduced Bees,* Bee World, 96:2, 40-44, DOI: 10.1080/0005772X.2019.1571211
- Agussalim and Agus A 2022 *Production of Honey, pot-pollen and propolis from Indonesian stingless bee Tetragonula laeviceps and the physicochemical properes of Honey: A review.* Livestock Research for Rural Development. Volume 34, Article #66. Retrieved April 18, 2023, from http://www.lrrd.org/lrrd34/8/3466alia.html
- Djakaria, S. A., et al., 2020 *Antioxidant and Antibacterial Activity of Selected Indonesian Honey against Bacteria of Acne* Jurnal Kimia Sains dan Aplikasi 23 (8) (2020): 267-275 https://doi.org/10.14710/jksa.23.8.267-275
- Octaviani, W., et al., 2020 Quality test comparison for *Wallacetrigona incisa* and *Tetragonula biroi* honey in Mappedeceng District, North Luwu Regency, South Sulawesi Province. Advances in Environmental Biology, 14(10): 1-8. DOI:10.22587/aeb.2020.14.10.1

Pollen & Chocolate

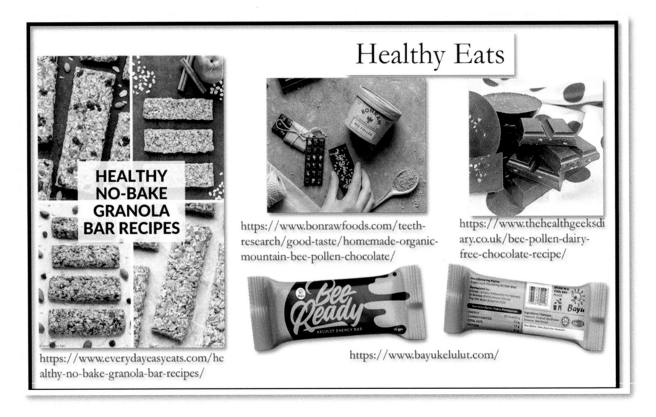

Figure 21 Pollen based products with honey or chocolate

Energy. Bee pollen can give a strong Burst of energy for a 3 pm slump because of its high levels of B vitamins. Benefits are Smooth Skin. ... Reduced Allergies. ... Immune Support. ... Normalize Cholesterol.

Source: https://www.magicmayan.com/index.php/2015/07/18/bee-pollen-the-superfood/

Here's what the research says about bee pollen benefits:

Relieving inflammation. ... Working as an antioxidant. ... Boosting liver health. ... Strengthening the immune system. ... Working as a dietary supplement. ... Easing symptoms of menopause. ... Reducing stress. ... Speeding healing. Source: https://www.healthline.com/health/bee-pollen-benefits%23research-says4

5

S.B. Product Types in ASEAN region.

- Meliponiculture and Apiculture
- Wild SB Honey and Honeybees
- Farmed Monoculture Nectar
- Maceration & Infusion
- Product derivatives & concoctions

Misconceptions and Misinterpretation by Region or Ethnic Cultures

In regions where the variety of Meliponines is limited and where the volume of harvestable raw Honey is just sufficient for domestic consumption, the idea of composing new processes and products is rather redundant, however, in areas where the variety of species is abundant and where certain taste rise as favourable, the unfavourable, like astringent honey, find new compositions and innovations of alternative ways of marketing the unfavourable tastes.

In Malaysia, Thailand and Indonesia, where such sour kinds of honey abound, especially the Dipterocarp-dependent ones, new mixes, macerations and infusion processes are born. In The Philippines, not many macerations appear as the *Tetragonula* spp. found there has little production and is not very keen on commercial; composition innovation. What we do find is honey mixed with coconut water, which is abundant. The bees are mainly used for pollination in coconut farms and Mango farms.

In the Middle East, Honey types and concoctions were initially done with Honeybees honey until many Islamic Regions like Pakistan, Bangladesh and South East Asian Countries with their influences started using Meliponine Honey instead of Apis Honey.

Indonesian 'Manuka' (*Leptospermum javanicum*) honey

Leptospermum is a genus of shrubs and small trees in the Myrtle family Myrtaceae commonly known as tea trees. Source: https://en.wikipedia.org/wiki/Leptospermum

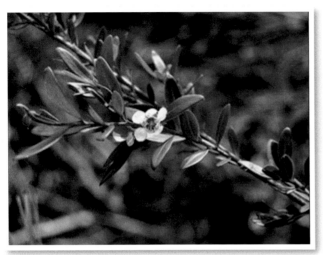 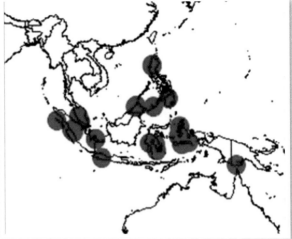

Leptospermum javanicum is a species of tree native to western and central Malesia. It has fibrous bark on the trunk, leaves much paler on the lower surface, relatively large white flowers[9] and woody fruit. Isolates from *L. javanicum* have shown potential as anti-cancer treatments by inducing apoptosis in lung cancer cells and distorting their ability to undergo metastasis.

The real N.Z. Manuka[10] has similar-looking white flowers and is often misrepresented in Indonesia.

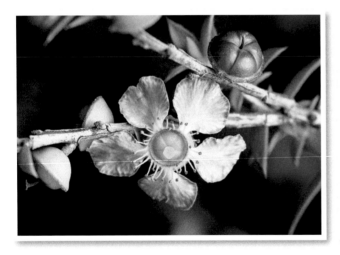 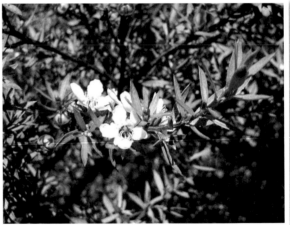

Figure 24 Pink Teatree (Leptospermum squarrosum)   *Figure 25 Manuka (Leptospermum scoparium) flowers.*

Manggis (Mangosteen) Honey & Propolis vs Tualang

- *Koompassia excelsa* (known as **Tualang** in Peninsula Malaysia, *tapang* in Sarawak, *mangaris* in Sabah, and *bangris* in Kalimantan) is found in Indonesia, Malaysia, the Philippines, and Thailand. Wild *Koompasia* honey by *Apis dorsata* in Malaysia is called **Tualang** honey.
- Other than *Koompasia* sp., trees honey from *A. dorsata* is **Uray** or **Sialang** Honey in Java. (Incidentally, see *ooray* on p. 59 on Davidson's Sour Plum - an Australian aborigine term))

---

9   https://en.wikipedia.org/wiki/Leptospermum_javanicum#/media/File:Leptosp_javan_160623-60110_tpl.JPG
10   https://en.wikipedia.org/wiki/Leptospermum_scoparium#/media/File:Manukaflowers.jpg

- **Manggis** (*K. excelsa*) is the tallest tree species in the Philippines (Located in Palawan). Honey produced by *A. dorsata* here is called **Manggis** Honey
- *Menggeris* (*K. excelsa*) in Indonesia…
- **Manggis** Honey in Malaysia is from SB under **Mangosteen** trees (*Garcinia mangostana*) esp *Geniotrigona. thoracica* in Kedah N. Peninsula and in South Thailand
- **Mangkhut** (*Garcinia mangostana*) in Thailand is also known as the "Queen of Tropical Fruits."

References

1. Issaro et al., 2013 *"Stingless Bee Honey Ii: Qualitative and Quantitative Studies On Honey Produced By Three Stingless Bee Species Collected From A Mangosteen Garden In Chantaburi Province, Thailand,"* The Thai Journal of Pharmaceutical Sciences: Vol. 38: Iss. 0, Article 5. Available at: https://digital.car.chula.ac.th/tjps/vol38/iss0/5
2. Vongsak et al. 2015 *In vitro alpha-glucosidase inhibition and free-radical scavenging activity of propolis from Thai stingless bees in mangosteen orchard* 0102-695X/© 2015 Sociedade Brasileira de Farmacognosia. *http://dx.doi.org/10.1016/j.bjp.2015.07.004*
3. Chewchinda & Vongsak, 2019 *Development and validation of a high-performance thin layer chromatography method for the simultaneous quantitation of α- and γ-mangostins in Thai stingless bee propolis* Revista Brasileira de Farmacognosia 29 (2019) 333–338
4. Asmara, W.H., & Nurlia, A., 2019. *Sialang Honey: Potency, Productivity, and Management in Musi Banyuasin (Case in Lubuk Bintialo Village, Musi Banyuasin Regency, South Sumatra)* Advances in Biological Sciences Research, volume 8

Local Misconceptions

1. Acacia Honey

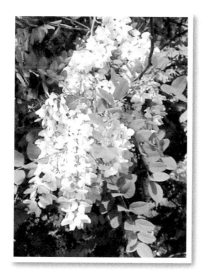

Figure 26 Robinia pseudoacacia flower, aka black locust

Original Acacia Honey from False Acacia

- In France, the acacia is the real name of the black locust. https://www.miel-factory.com/en/blogs/blog/recolte-miel-acacia The "Acacia honey" collected is highly sought after because it is very fine, tasteless, transparent and slowly crystallizes. It must be extracted as soon as the flowering is over to avoid the "pollution" of other honeydews, which clouds the product.
- Nigerian "Acacia honey" is derived from the nectar of the *Robinia pseudoacacia* flower, also known as the black locust or **false acacia tree** of Nigeria[11].

---

[11] https://pubmed.ncbi.nlm.nih.gov/26709666/https://doi.org/10.1080/14786419.2014.940945

- As per Nuru et al., 2016, Pollination ecology, nectar secretion dynamics, and honey production potentials of *Acacia ehrenbergiana* (Hayne) and *Acacia tortilis* (Forsk.) Hayne, Leguminosae (Mimosoideae), in an arid region of Saudi Arabia, the flowers are visited by bees which make "Acacia Honey" from the nectar.
- Acacia Honey as a supplementary diet has been shown to lower blood pressure, increase haemoglobin levels, and lower the risk of heart disease, stroke, and some types of cancer[12] (including lung cancer).
- Acacia Honey may also be used to prevent and treat acne. Its strong antibacterial activity could help keep your skin bacteria-free, which may improve or prevent common skin conditions like acne. Source[13]

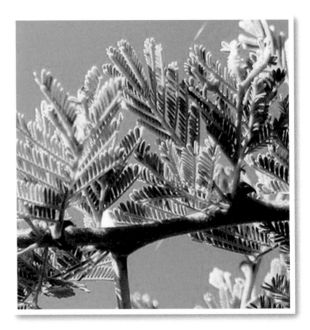

Figure 27 Acacia tortilis (Forsk.) Hayne (Wikimedia)

- *A. mangium* was planted in Sabah in 1976 (Udarbe & Hepburn 1986), and a decade later, there was approximately 21,100 ha of it[14].

The Myth of *Acacia mangium* Honey

- In SE Asia, the preferred provision for Bee farms is *Acacia Mangium*. Introduced in Sabah in 1976, A. mangium was widely planted for its valued importance in the paper pulp industries.
- Newspaper conglomerates now look to bee farming to complement their reduction of paper requirements, and *A. mangium* is a robust growing species and flowers profusely all year round and, in addition, provides for leaf petiole nectar
- However, this EFN gives insufficient electroconductivity, inevitably disqualifying S.B. honey in the Codex Alimentarius.

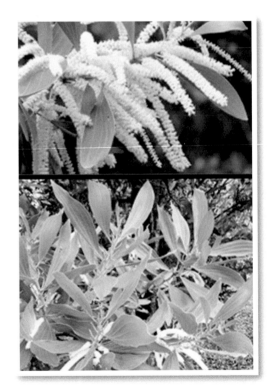

Figure 28 Black Wattle (A. mangium)

---

12 https://www.eatingwell.com/article/7956509/carbs-you-should-be-buying-for-better-blood-pressure/

13 https://beebudzhq.com/articles/3-local-honey-that-can-only-be-found-in-malaysia/#:~:text=The%20Kelulut%20honey%20gets%20its,nutritious%20compared%20ordinary%20natural%20honey.

14 Lee, S. S. (2018). Observations On The Successes And Failures Of Acacia Plantations In Sabah And Sarawak And The Way Forward. Journal of Tropical Forest Science, 30(5), 468.

Acacia honey from Indonesia

Acacia crassicarpa[15] (northern wattle, thick-podded salwood, brown salwood, Papua New Guinea red wattle, red wattle; syn. *Racosperma crassicarpum* (A.Cunn. ex Benth.) Pedley.) is a tree native to Australia (Queensland), West Papua (Indonesia) and Papua New Guinea.

One of the main products of the people of Jambi is known to be honey, specifically acacia honey[16]. Like most honey, acacia honey is widely consumed and has health benefits. Acacia honey has a dark colour and a floral scent with a sweet, soft, and slightly bitter taste. Acacia honey is rich in antioxidants, one of which is flavonoids. According to research, foods that contain high levels of flavonoids can reduce the risk of chronic disease.

The Industrial Plantation Forest (HTI) concession area, with many acacia trees, is the right place to start honey bee cultivation. While the trunks of *Acacia crassicarpa* trees are used as the raw material for making paper, the nectar from the flowers is the food source for acacia honey bees, the superior bee Apis mellifera. Interestingly, *Acacia crassicarpa* trees can only grow on peatlands, actively driving the community to participate in peat conservation.

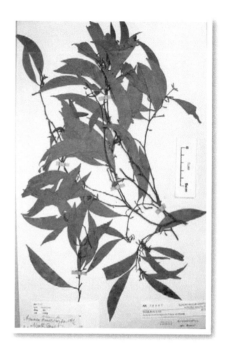

Figure 29 Acacia crassicarpa

This potential prompted PT Wirakarya Sakti (WKS), one of the business units of APP Sinar Mas, to start focusing on honey bee cultivation as part of the DMPA program in 2020. Pak Wanudin, a senior farmer in honey bee cultivation. As one of the Champion Farmers who is a role model for other honey farmers, Wanudin's acacia honey sales volume has reached 7 tons a month. After two years since he began honey bee cultivating, he has doubled his profits. His products have also expanded to Batam Island and is now entering the Singaporean and Malaysian market.

Since partnering with PT WKS' DMPA program, Wanudin has experienced many economic changes for himself and his group. Now the group is focused on sharing the partnership profits and has other income from bee cultivation to help sustain their income.

15 https://en.wikipedia.org/wiki/Acacia_crassicarpa#/media/File:Acacia_crassicarpa_A. Cunn._ex_Benth._(AM_AK75557).jpg

16 https://asiapulppaper.com/-/the-sweet-story-behind-acacia-honey

Seagrape Honey (of Florida)[17]

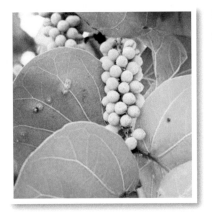

Figure 30 Seagrape honey is from Coccoloba uvifera flowers

Seagrape honey is honey produced by bees foraging *Coccoloba uvifera* flowers. It has a light colour and delicate flavour, making it an excellent choice for desserts or drinks, but you can also use it on toast or as part of your morning oatmeal.

However, in the *Asia-Pacific region, Seaprapes (Caulerpa lentillifera)* ulvophyte green algae from coastal regions. A delicacy sometimes consumed as a salad and dressed with honey.

- In Sabah (*Latok*), Korea (*bada podo*), Philippines (*latô* or *arosep*), Bali (*bulung)* Japan (*umi-budo* or *kubiretsuta*), Vietnam (*rong nho* or *rong nho biển*), Singapore & Riau (as *latoh*)

- It is this dish that is often confused with the original Seagrape honey

Honey & Herbal Integration

Nutmeg (*Myristica fragrans*) honey

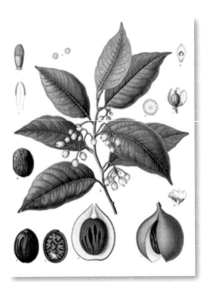

Figure 31 Nutmeg Plant

Nutmeg[18] is extensively used in several Ayurvedic medicines and formulations to promote sexual health. Nutmeg butter, a fat derived from the seed, is used in perfumery and toothpaste. Applying Nutmeg powder, honey, or milk on your skin helps control excess oil and removes pigmentation[19].

Nutmeg powder[20] can be consumed with a teaspoonful of honey and mixed in fruit juices, amla juice and milk products.

Contains powerful antioxidants... Has anti-inflammatory properties. ...May boost libido. ...Has antibacterial properties. ...

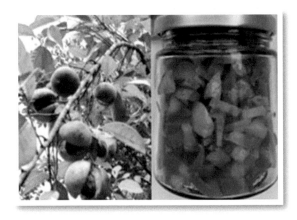

Figure 32 Honey-soaked nutmeg fruit isa candied fruit snack

---

17 https://worldofoney.com/2022/02/20/sea-grape-honey-the-sweet-ingredient-with-a-surprising-history/#:~:text=The%20sweetener%20was%20first%20used,because%20of%20its%20antiseptic%20qualities.

18 https://en.wikipedia.org/wiki/Myristica_fragrans#/media/File:Myristica_fragrans_-_K%C3%B6hler%E2%80%93s_Medizinal-Pflanzen-097.jpg

19 https://www.1mg.com/ayurveda/nutmeg-162

20 https://www.refreshyourlife.in/blog/nutmeg-powder-uses-benefits-and-recipes

The honey-soaked nutmeg fruit is one kind of candied fruit snack. Nutmeg fruit is peeled, sliced and soaked in honey for two weeks. The fleshy nutmeg slices absorb honey and taste unique. Honey-soaked nutmeg fruit helps in digestion and is a good relief for gastric problems.

Cinnamon Flower Honey

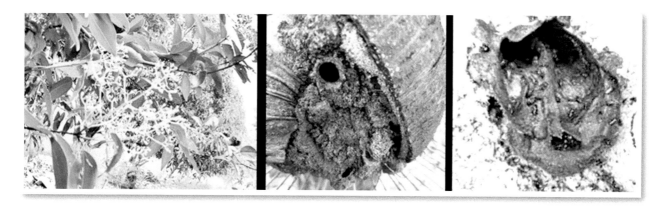

Figure 33 Cinnamon honey is produced by SB in Organic Cinnamon farms

Lowers risk of heart disease. A cinnamon honey concoction is very helpful in reducing cholesterol levels. ...Boosts immunity. ...Used for treating skin infections. ...Helps Strengthen Joints. ...Good for diabetes. ...Treats bladder infections. ...Helps with stomach disorders. ...Gets rid of bad breath[21][22].

References:

- Rao, P.V. & Gan, S.H. 2014 Cinnamon: a multifaceted medicinal plant. *Evid Based Complement Alternat Med. 2014;2014:642942. doi: 10.1155/2014/642942.*
- Fuentes et al. 2010 Antioxidant and Antibacterial Properties of Crude Methanolic Extracts of Cinnamomum mercadoi Vidal *Phil J of Nat Sci 15 (2010): 9-15*
- Femine, C. P. G. 2018 Efficacy of cinnamon in the treatment of orofacial conditions. *Int J Contemp Dent Med Rev, vol.2018, Article ID: 020918, 2018. doi: 10.15713/ins.ijcdmr.130*
- Anand, V. 2016 Cinnamomum zeylanicum Linn. The spice with multi potential *Systematic Reviews in Pharmacy., 2016;7(1):24-29*

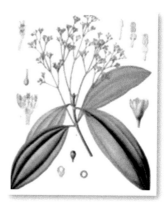

Figure 34 Cinnamomum sp. (Wikipedia)

Cinnamon Infused Honey

- Cinnamon (Cinnamomum zeylanicum) from Sri Lanka is infused in Stingless bee Honey
- It may help support blood sugar control, protect against heart disease, and reduce inflammation[23].

---

21 https://xedogo.duenews.dynu.net/q-and-a/what-disease-does-cinnamon-cure
22 Ref: Devi, N., et al, 2021, Herbal Medicine for Urinary Tract Infections with the Blazing Nanotechnology, Journal of Nanoscience and Nanotechnology, Vol. 21, 3495–3512.
23 https://www.healthline.com/nutrition/10-proven-benefits-of-cinnamon

- The flavour of the Philippine cinnamon is minty and warm, while the flavour of the Philippine stingless bee honey is fruity.

Cinnamon Tea[24] + Honey

In the Philippines, *C. anacardium, C. panayense, C. inners, C. mindanaense & C. philippinense* Tea recipes:

1. Boil 300 ml water. Lower fire.;
2. Drop 1-2 Philippine cinnamon chips and Simmer for 5-8 mins.;
3. Tips - air dry only the bark (do not dry in full sun), and simmer in a low fire when brewing.;
4. Add one tablespoon of stingless bee honey.
5. For stomachaches (from diarrhoea, flatulence, indigestion, etc.),

Pepper Elder (*Peperomia pellucida*) Honey

- *Peperomia pellucida*, Pepper Elder, locally known as 'sinaw-sinaw' in the Philippines (literally 'shining') or 'sireh cina' in Malay
- *P. pellucida* has been used for treating abdominal pain, abscesses, acne, boils, colic, fatigue, gout, headache, renal disorders, and rheumatic joint pain[25].

Peperomia pellucida (sinaw-sinaw) extract, a fleshy herb plant commonly found in the Philippines, is believed to treat UTI ((urinary tract disorder or infections) in traditional folk medicine

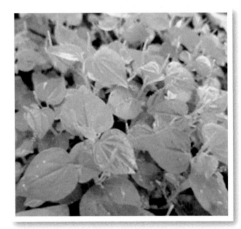

Figure 35 Pepper Elder (Peperomia pellucida)

Salam Infused Honey

- *Vachellia flava*, synonym *Acacia ehrenbergiana*, is a species of drought-resistant bush or small tree, commonly known as **salam** in Arabic.
- In the 60s, Malay Haj pilgrims brought back Salam Honey (*Acacia ehrenbergiana*)
- Malay cuisine included Salam (West Indian Bay leaves) for aroma and meat tenderizing.
- Wild Honey was infused with Salam (*Pimento racemose*) for flavour and fragrance.

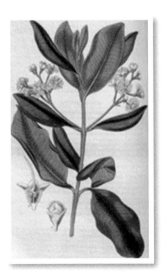

Figure 36 Salam leaves

---

24 Recipe by November G. Canieso-Yeo, Plantsville Health, Bacolod City, Negros Occidental, Visayas (novembercanieso@gmail.com

25 https://positivepsychology.org.ng/health-benefits-of-peperomia-pellucida-shining-bush-or-pepper-elder

CHAPTER 6

Fruit Farms, Orchards and Plantations

Sweet Coconut Honey (Nam Wan Honey)

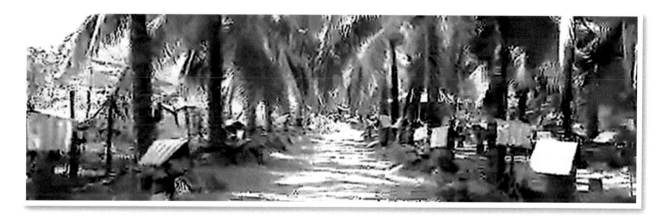

Figure 37 Kelapa Pandan farm 9Fragrant coconut cultivar) with meliponiculture in Langkawi, Malaysia

- Langkawi Pandan Coconut (Green Dwarf) Plantation ★Nam Wan (Sweet Green Dwarf cultivar) The Honey has a rich, fruity flavour
- Muar, Johor Kelapa Gading/Mawar *Cocos nucifera* L. Dwarf var. (Nana) /Malayan Dwarf
- Fragrant Coconut – *Cocos nucifera* L. [Aromatic Dwarf] in Thailand Fragrant coconut, or Ma-Phrao Nam-Hom in the Thai language
- Namwan means Nectar in Thai – Soak ginger and lemons overnight in coconut water, then sweeten with honey.

Coconut water, Sap or Vinegar & Honey – available in the Philippines

Health Benefits of Coconut Water and Honey: – Promote healthy skin and prevents premature ageing… Strengthens the immune system… Boosts energy… Helps with digestion… Lowers blood sugar levels… Good for the kidneys… Enhances cardiovascular health.

In the Philippines, *Botung* for coconut water, *Tuba* is newly harvested coconut sap... the daily harvest. *Tuba* is at least 12 hrs in the aerobic or open-air... *Bahal* for week-old coconut sap. *Bahalina* has fermented anaerobically. Vinegar is *Suka* (Malay= *cuka*) in Visayan and Tagalog, while Langgaw is an Ilonggo Term for Vinegar.

Langgaw, in Visayan Terms, is stagnant water. Spicy Vinegar in Ilonggo is *Sinamak, Pinakurat* in Iligan and *Kusisang* in Zamboanga and Bohol. *Langgaw* for fermented, months to year-old coconut sap. a.k.a. vinegar. At any of these stages, they may be mixed with honey as a drink: 2 Tbsp. Honey +1 Tbsp. Apple cider or coconut vinegar+ one glass of lukewarm water removes respiratory (COVID) symptoms and even alleviates kidney stones. (Mindanao home-remedy)

Coconut vinegar, derived from fermented coconut sap, is rich in probiotics and acetic acid that can help support a healthy gut. This vinegar has a lighter, sweeter flavour than apple cider vinegar, and you can easily substitute it in recipes that call for ACV.

Lychee (*Litchi chinensis*) Honey

Lychee is a great source of dietary fibre, protein, proanthocyanins and polyphenolic compounds, which makes it an energizing fruit. 'Lychee Honey' is helpful in digestive issues and cognitive disorders, helping improve blood circulation and protecting the body from various diseases and afflictions.

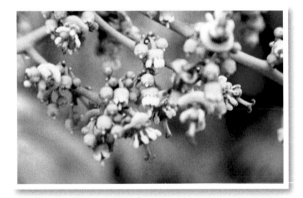

Pure Lychee Honey is made with nectar from bees from lychee orchards in Thailand. Lychee Honey is a light-yellow honey that is mild, minty and has slight hints of Lychee after-taste.

Lychee honey is rich in vitamins and minerals; abundant vitamin C in lychee boosts the immune system and helps heal wounds and repair. Lychee honey is proven effective in improving bone health, especially in women and children.

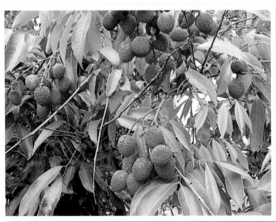

Figure 38 Lychee (Litchi chinensis)

Rambutan (*Nephelium lappaceum*) **Honey**

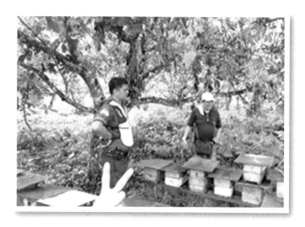

- Available in the Philippines and Thailand, although in Malaysia, Rambutan is planted with Calamansi (*Citrus madurensis*, the Calamondin) in Meliponaries to ensure the bees have other forage sources when the rambutan season is over.
- Rambutan Honey from Thailand -Winner of a Honey Ranking event during the Int. Meliponine Conf 2016
- Rambutan trees interspersed with Calamansi Trees to provide sources inter rambutan season in Selangor, Malaysia
- Yuslianti, E.R., et al., 2016, Effect of Rambutan Honey (*Nephelium lappaceum*) Acute Administration on Mortality, Body Weight, Toxicity Symptoms and Relative Organ Weight of Swiss Websters Mice. Research Journal of Toxins, 8: 1-7. DOI: 10.3923/rjt.2016.1.7

Pitaya (*Selenicereus undatus*) **Honey**

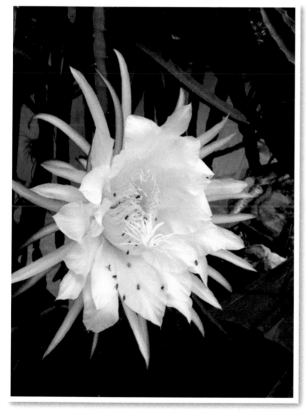

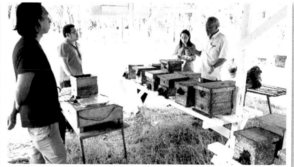

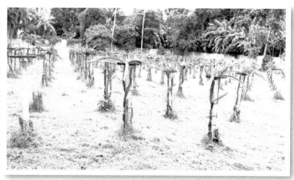

Figure 40 Meliponiculture with Pitaya (Seleniferous undatus). Dragon fruit farm in CvSU

- Model Meliponary in The CvSU campus Dragon Fruit farm in Cavite
- The sweet and tart flavour of the Dragon Fruit (Magenta flesh) is perfectly balanced with the sweetness of the honey, creating a unique flavour.
- Macerated Dragon fruit (white flesh) and the infused honey's flavour profile are floral, fruity, and citrus.

- Dragon Fruit Health Benefits: It's rich in antioxidants like flavonoids, phenolic acid, and betacyanin. ... It's naturally fat-free and high in fibre. ... It may help lower your blood sugar. ... It contains prebiotics, which are foods that feed the healthy bacteria called probiotics in your gut. ... It can strengthen your immune system[26],[27].

Pili Nut (*Canarium ovatum*) **Honey & Resin**

- Pili resin is known as "Manila Elemi", which is used for pharmaceutical products, colours, varnish, ointments, and perfumes
- Anti-microbes, fungi or viruses in minor wounds and cuts. Elemi oils contain natural antiseptic and analgesic properties that help eliminate bacteria and protect against infection. Powerful as a healing tonic, Elemi oil's anti-inflammatory properties[28] also help reduce aches and pains.
- The Health Benefits of Pili Nuts: They Fight Inflammation. ... Lower LDL Cholesterol. ... Have Antioxidant-driven Properties. ... They Enhance Your Regeneration. ...They Strengthen Your Bones. ... They Help You Keep Your Brain in Shape.

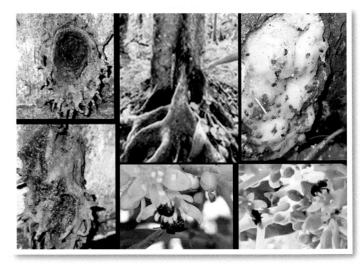

Figure 41 Tetragonula biroi nest entrance at Pili Nut tree & Resin of the Pili nut (Canarium ovatum)

Avocado (*Persea americana*) Honey

Avocado nectar provides honey with a rich source of Iron, B vitamins and phenolic compounds, such as flavonoids. This honey has traditionally been used for its diuretic properties, helping us to eliminate water from the body and electrolytes that remain in our body stored.

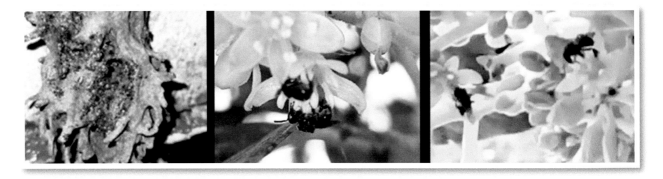

Figure 42 Tetragonula biroi nest entrance at Avocado (Persea americana)

26   https://github.com/scottschmidl/Fruits-and-Veggies-Nutrition-Facts/blob/master/data/nutri_facts_name.csv
27   https://baybowlsme.com/
28   https://www.edensgarden.com/blogs/news/top-elemi-essential-oil-uses-benefits

Avocado honey benefits your digestive system and immune system[29]. It heals your skin, cuts, allergies, and more! It's a tasty treat, especially if you like honey, and it only has 64 calories per tablespoon.

Mango (*Mangifera indica*) Blossom Honey

100% Pure Honey from Mango Flowers.
Health Benefits

- Has antibacterial and antifungal properties.
- It may aid in healing minor burns, wounds and ulcers.
- Helps with detoxing the body and resolving gastrointestinal issues such as constipation.
- It may help ease coughs, flu, sore throats, sinus and asthma.

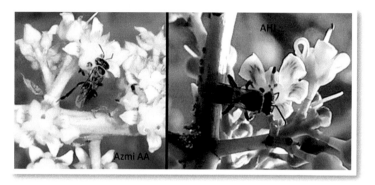

Figure 43 Two types of Mango flowers favoured by Meliponines.

Other forms are young Mango flesh macerated with honey is a favourite snack with high fibre content. One 3/4 serving of these superfruits contains seven percent of your daily fibre requirements.

Sunflower (*Helianthus annuus*) honey and Sunflower seed honey roasted

- Raw sunflower honey is considered one of nature's true superfoods, and it plays an important role as an antioxidant, anti-inflammatory and antibacterial agent. With a range of health-boosting metabolites, raw sunflower honey can be considered a healthier alternative to sweeten food and drinks.
- Sunflower honey is usually floral but can be with honeydew impurities, which change its colour to darker. Sunflowers bloom very late when no other flower sources of nectar, and bees often fly away for some honeydew into nearby vegetation.
- Raw sunflower honey should consist of above 45% sunflower pollen. The honey created by bees which have primarily collected the nectar from sunflower fields, is defined by its: High level of glucose and fructose, low glucose/fructose ratio & low level of sucrose.
- Sunflower seeds may help lower blood pressure, cholesterol and blood sugar as they contain vitamin E, magnesium, protein, linoleic fatty acids and several plant compounds[30].

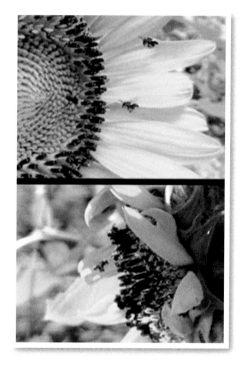

Figure 44 Sunflower seeds & SB on Helianthus annuus

---

29 https://niftywellness.com/avocado-honey-benefits/
30 https://www.healthline.com/nutrition/sunflower-seeds

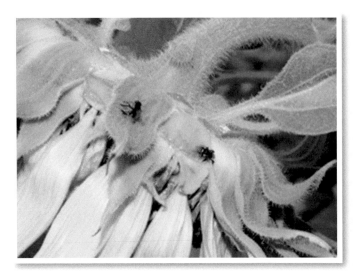
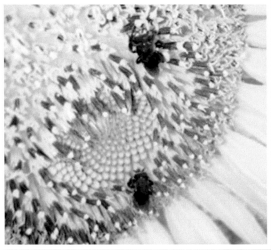

Figure 45 Sunflower (Helianthus annuus)

Sunflower (*Helianthus annuus*) seeds

Sunflower seed: The showy outer ray petals help attract pollinators. Bees go from flower to flower within the disc, becoming covered with pollen. They then pollinate[31] other sunflowers as they go from plant to plant. The success of sunflowers as a crop for seeds and oil depends totally on bees.

References

- Chambo, E., Garcia, R., de Oliverira, N. T., & Doarte-Junior, J. (2011). *Honey bee visitation to sunflower effects on pollination and plant genotype.* Sci, Aqric. (Piracic).
- Cimu, I. (1960). *Results of bee pollination of Sunflowers.* Apicultura. 33(1) :, 18-20.
- Morgado, L., Carvalho, C., Souza, B., & Santana, M. (2002). Fauna of bees (Hymenoptera: Apoidea) on sunflower flowers, *Helianthus annuus* L., in Lavras-MG Ciencia. Agrotecnologia 26: (in Portuguese, with abstract in English)., 1167-1177.
- Orstratrat, O. (1993). *The role of honey bees, certinini bees and stingless bees on sunflower (Helianthus annus L.) pollination.* Ms. thesis. Kasetsart University.
- Rajasri, M., Kana Kadurga, K., Durqa Rani, V., & Anuradha, C. (2012). *Honey Bees- potential pollinators in hybrid seed production of Sunflower.* International Journal of Applied Biology and Pharmaceutical Technology, 3(2): 216-221.
- Sawatthum, A., Tonwitoowat, R., & Umnuaysit, K. (2017). *The Role Of Stingless Bee And European Honey Bee In Pollination Of Confectionery Sunflower.* Bangkok: AKM-IMS3C.
- Singh, M., Singh, & Devi, C. (1998). *Foraging behaviour of Apis cerana himalaga on Sunflower and rape seed. In Asian Bees and Beekeeping Progress of Research and Development,* Proceeding of Fourth Asian Apicaltural Association International Conference, Kathmandu. March 23 – 28, 1998., 199-202.
- Somnuk. (1990). *Bees pollinate the Sunflower.* Housing Agriculture 14 (6): 97 – 103.
- Teixeira, L., & Zampieron, S. (2008). (2008). *Phenology, floral biology studies of the Sunflower (Helianthus annuus, Compositae) and associated flower visitors in different year seasons.* Ciência et Práxis 1: 5-14 (in Portuguese, with abstract in English).

31 https://homeguides.sfgate.com/bees-pollinate-sunflowers-65431.html

CHAPTER 7

Dominant Tree species Forests

Gelam (*Melaleuca cajaputi*) Honey – a.k.a. Paperbark, Kayu Puteh

- Great Farm in Sg. Jang, KKB, Selangor, Malaysia has an acre simulacra of *Melaleuca cajaputi* with 50 hives of *Heterotrigona itama*. Originally planned for harvesting of Cajuputi (Kayu Puteh) oil. The "bee air" in this simulacrum has relieving properties for bronchial ailments (Pers. obs.)

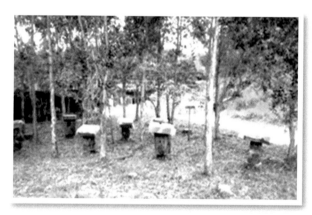

Figure 46 Stingless bee culture in a Gelam Simulacra

References:

- Putri Shuhaili S. et al., 2016, Gelam Honey: A Review of Its Antioxidant, Anti-inflammatory, Anti-cancer and Wound Healing Aspects Med & Health 2016;11(2): 105-116 https://doi.org/10.17576/MH.2016.1102.01
- Mohd Kamal, D.A. et al. Physicochemical and Medicinal Properties of Tualang, Gelam and Kelulut Honeys: A Comprehensive Review. Nutrients 2021, 13, 197. https://doi.org/10.3390/nu13010197
- Johari et al., 2019: A review on biological activities of Gelam honey Journal of Applied Biology & Biotechnology 2019;7(01):71-78 DOI: 10.7324/JABB.2019.70113

Peculiar Honey in Indonesia[32]

- Clover honey has a great taste that's ideal for baking and having on toast from clover blossoms (genus Trifolium) may be confused with Clove Infused Honey
- Uray Honey – *Apis Dorsata* (forest bees). This honey contains various flower essences that maintain healthy digestion and endurance, nourish the skin, and increase nutrient intake. a.k.a Sialang Honey
- Calliandra honey – by honey bees raised in the Calliandra forest area. *Calliandra calothyrsus,* introduced to Indonesia in 1936, was adopted by Javanese farmers for fuel-wood production and land reclamation.
- Sumbawa forest honey – thick texture and low water content *Bidara* tree or *Ziziphus mauritiana*
- Manuka honey (*Leptospermum scoparium*) Some S.B. keepers provide an alternative species, *Leptospermum javanicum,* in their Meliponaries.

Clover Honey

Keep your brain healthy. Clover honey contains compounds that produce hydrogen peroxide, which can help to kill bacteria and prevent infections. It may also be effective as a topical antibacterial dressing for wounds such as foot ulcers. The phenolic acid in clover honey may help to protect brain health[33].

Clover (*Trifolium repens)* honey is a thick, sweet syrup made by bees that collect the nectar of clover plants. It's mild in taste and light in colour, making it a popular choice among honey enthusiasts[34].

Red clover (*Trifolium pratense)* blooms in the morning. The photo was taken in the hills of Rembangan in Jember, East Java, Indonesia.

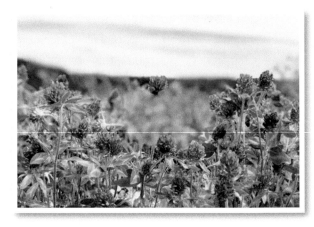

Figure 47 Red clover (Trifolium pratense)

Clover honey is high in flavanols, antioxidants that can help to regulate your blood pressure, which in turn helps to protect your heart health. Flavanol content also leads to better blood flow[35] and transportation of oxygen and nutrients throughout your body. Source: https://www.webmd.com/

32 https://voi.id/en/lifestyle/39896#:~:text=The%20name%20uray%20honey%20is,directly%20even%20without%20being%20processed.

33 https://www.webmd.com/diet/health-benefits-clover-honey

34 https://www.healthline.com/nutrition/clover-honey

35 https://www.webmd.com/diet/health-benefits-clover-honey

Calliandra Honey

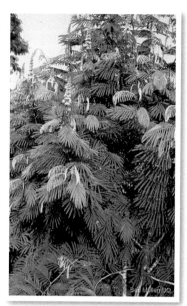

- Calliandra was introduced into Indonesia from Guatemala in 1936 when foresters carried two seed samples to Java.
- Kaliandra honey improves testosterone levels, diameter and epithelial thickness of seminiferous tubule of white rats (Rattus norvegicus) due to malnutrition ...
- Ismawati, R. - (2018) *The Effects of Kaliandra Honey (Calliandra calothyrsus) on Oxygen Saturation (SPO2) In Rats Exposed To Physical Stress.* International Journal of Public Health and Clinical Sciences[36], 5 (5). pp. 210-217. ISSN 2289-7577
- Merlina, P. – (2016) *The Effect of Honey Harvesting Time on Kaliandra Plant Area (Calliandra calothyrsus) to The Production, Moisture, Viscosity and Sugar Content* April Jurnal Ilmu dan Teknologi Hasil Ternak 11(1):46-51 DOI:10.21776/ ub.jitek.2016.011.01.1.5

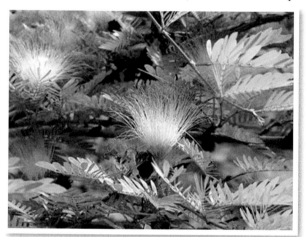

Figure 48 Calliandra calothyrsus in a Meliponary in South Kalimantan

- Malaysian Stingless Bee keepers favour the more available *Calliandra surinamensis* (Powder Puff Plant)

Figure 49 Calliandra surinamensis

Ziziphus (Bidara) honey

Another honey native to Indonesia and famous for a long time is the forest honey of Sumbawa. Its trademark is a thick texture and low water content compared to other honey. Sumbawa's dry and hot natural conditions also affect honey yields. Sumbawa forest honey is produced by bees that take nectar from the *Bidara* tree or *Ziziphus mauritiana*.

Therefore, it is recommended to use Ziziphus honey as a natural preservative and antibacterial agent. Also, it could potentially be used as a therapeutic agent against bacterial infection, particularly the tested microorganisms.

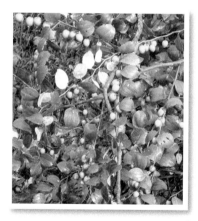

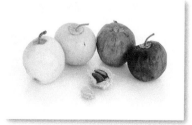

Figure 50 Bidara tree or Ziziphus mauritiana.

---

36 Lim, P. (2019). Systematic review on the prevalence of illness and stress and their associated risk factors among educators in Malaysia. PLoS One, 14(5), e0217430.

References:

- Nairfana, M., et al., 2022, Variability of secondary metabolites from leaves of Ziziphus mauritiana obtained from different locations in Sumbawa, Indonesia BIODIVERSITAS Volume 23, Number 9, September 2022 Pages: 4948-4957 DOI: 10.13057/biodiv/d230965
- Alqarni, A.S., 2015, Honeybee Foraging, Nectar Secretion, and Honey Potential of Wild Jujube Trees, Ziziphus nummularia. Neotrop Entomol 44, 232–241 (2015). https://doi.org/10.1007/s13744-015-0279-4
- Ekhtelat, M., et al., Effect of Iranian Ziziphus honey on the growth of some foodborne pathogens J Nat Sci Biol Med. 2016 Jan-Jun; 7(1): 54–57. doi: 10.4103/0976-9668.175069

CHAPTER 8

Honey Macerations

Traditional methods by the villagers

- The Sea Cucumber (Gamat (Actinopyga sp.) It is cleaned, and the stomach is removed, then cleaned and evaporated into honey. After two weeks, chopped and then put back into honey and can be used for medical purposes or as a supplement.
- Garlic, ginger and lemon honey. These three ingredients are cooked and then cooled. Newly blended with honey and stored.
- Pepper Elder (*Peperomia pellucida*) & halba (Fenugreek) - whole plant & shoots washed and cleaned, then boiled with fenugreek, cooled and mixed with honey.
- Tongkat Ali's sweet honey (finely ground Eurycoma longifolia Jack and macerated in honey),
- Garlic honey. (Garlic is burned and soaked in honey for two weeks.)

Gamat Honey (Sea cucumber)

The Sea Cucumber [*Gamat* (Actinyga sp.)] The most popular remedy here in Langkawi Island, Malaysia, is for the problem of spinal disorders, waist/back problems, and urinary tract, and. The body is quite lethargic, and the effects on the body are very noticeable after taking it, especially the system of swelling, which means increasing the body's metabolism rate[37].

Sea Cucumbers Honey

Sea Cucumbers in San Guillermo, Leyte Is., Visayas Philippines, are being supplied to Chinese Medicine Halls in Manila, where some are macerated in honey. Commonly known by various names in local dialects, such as "balat", "balatan", "ba–at", and "bat."

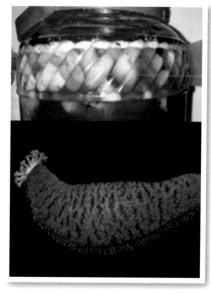

Figure 51 Honey Maceration of Brown Sea cucumber (or "deep-water redfish"), Actinopyga echinites. Gamat

---

37 Reference:
Haryanto et al., 2017 A prospective observational study using sea cucumber and honey as topical therapy for diabetic foot ulcers in Indonesia. Journal of Wellness and Health Care Vol. 41 (2) 41-56

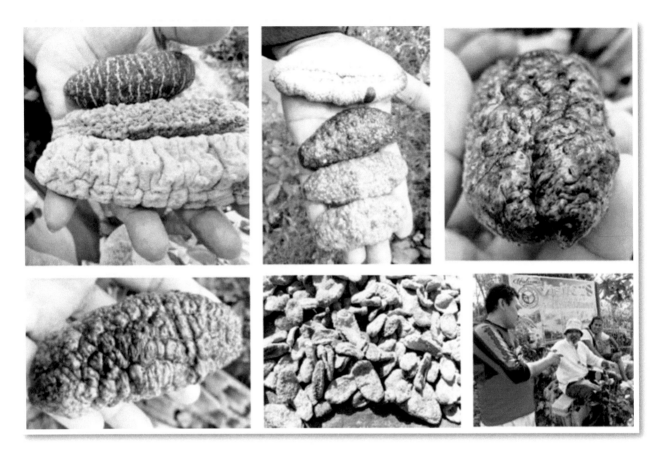

Figure 52 Sea Cucumbers: San Guillermo is a fishing village with the main commodity Sea cucumbers.

Suggested maceration recipe in honey practised in Langkawi Island, Malaysia:

- The Sea Cucumber (Gamat (Actinopyga sp.)) Is cleaned, and the stomach is removed, cleaned, and evaporated into honey.
- After two weeks, chopped and then put back into honey and can be used for medicinal purposes or as a supplement.
- The most popular here are the problem of spinal disorders, waist problems, and urinary tract, and the body is quite lethargic. The effects on the body are very noticeable after taking it, especially the system of swelling, which means increasing the body's metabolism rate.

References:

- Gerard, C., et al., n.d. *Herbal medicines for urinary tract infections – Global contemporary naturopathic herbal medicine practice and Balkan ethnopharmacology: A scoping review.* JBI Evidence Synthesis
- DOA, Rep. of Philippines, 2013, *Size regulation for sea cucumber collection and trade.* Bfar Administrative Circular No. 2. 4 8 Series Of 2013
- Schoppe, S., 2020, *Sea cucumber fishery in the Philippines* **S.P.C. Beche-de-mer Information Bulletin #13**

References on Sea cucumber health benefits in Indonesia

- Haryanto et al., 2017, *A prospective observational study using sea cucumber and honey as topical therapy for diabetic foot ulcers in Indonesia.* Journal of Wellness and Health Care Vol. 41 (2) 41-56.
- Adam, M, et a*l., 2022, The Benefits of Golden Sea Cucumber (Stichopus hermanni) as an Alternative Antimicrobial Material in Oral Health* Journal of International Dental and Medical Research ISSN 1309-100X Alternative Antimicrobial Material Volume · 15 · Number · 4 · 2022, Page 1806
- Haryanto, H., et al., *2022, Effect of Sea Cucumber on Reducing Periwound Maceration and Inflammation-Related Indicators in Patients With Diabetic Foot Ulcers Indonesia* Indonesian Nursing Journal of Education and Clinic (INJEC) Volume 7 Issue 1, Juni 2022 DOI: 10.24990/injec. v7i1.504

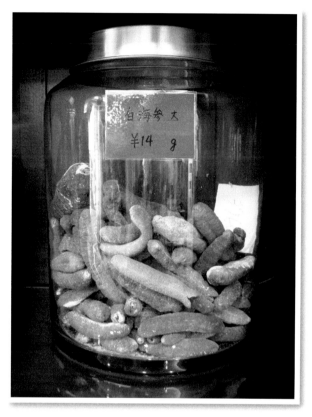

Figure 53 Jar of dried, gutted sea cucumbers at a traditional Chinese medicine emporium in Yokohama, Japan (Wikimedia)

- Azman et al., 2021, *AntioxidantActivity Synergy Between StinglessBee Honey and Sea Cucumber ExtractCombination for Food Supplement* Progress in Engineering Application and Technology Vol. 3 No. 1 (2021) p. 1-10
- Pangkey, H., 2012, *Prospect of Sea Cucumber Culture in Indonesia as Potential Food Sources.* Journal of Coastal Development Volume 15, Number 2, 114 - 124

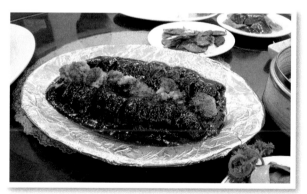

Figure 54 Sea cucumber dish (Wikipedia)

Dried Figs and Honey

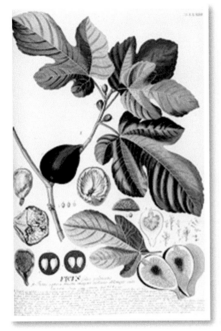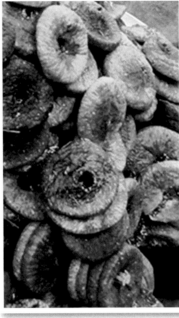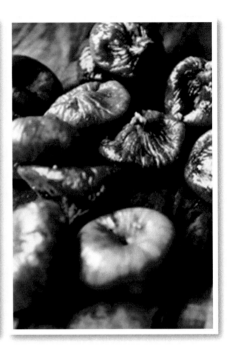

Figure 55 Left: Fig Plant (Ficus carica; Middle: QDried Figs; Right: Honey Macerated

Raw figs are 79% water, 19% carbohydrates, 1% protein, and contain negligible fat (table). They are a moderate source (14% of the Daily Value, DV) of dietary fibre and 310 kilojoules (74 kcal) of food energy per 100-gram serving and do not supply essential micronutrients in significant contents (table).

When dehydrated to 30% water, figs have a carbohydrate content of 64%, protein content of 3%, and fat content of 1%.[42] In a 100-gram serving, providing 1,041 kJ (249 kcal) of food energy, dried figs are a rich source (more than 20% DV) of dietary fibre and the essential mineral manganese (26% DV), while calcium, Iron, magnesium, potassium, and vitamin K are in moderate amounts[38].

Honey Macerated Dried Figs (*Ficus carica*)

- Honey Mixed Figs gives relief from sore throat.
- Honey and Figs have a high number of antioxidants and help digestion.
- The high amount of Fibre\s in Figs helps Clear Excess Cholesterol in the digestive system.
- Figs help Improve Haemoglobin levels as it has Iron, a key component of Haemoglobin.

---

38 https://en.wikipedia.org/wiki/Fig

Honey Macerated Miracle Berry (*Synsepalum dulcificum*)

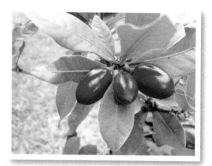

- *Synsepalum dulcificum* is also recognized as Miracle fruit, Miracle berry, and miraculous berry. It makes sour food taste sweet (Obafemi et al., 2019).
- Traditional healers in Johor, Malaysia, macerate these berries with sour honey and treat breast cancer patients. The berry itself has low sugar content.
- In Lombok, Indonesia, rural folk feed their cockerel this berry with honey to win cock fights.
- Some selected medicinal and magico-spiritual uses and applications of the miracle plant in Benin and Ghana.

References[39]:

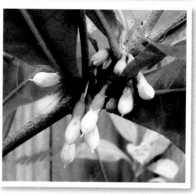

- Merriam, S. & Muhamad, M., 2013, *Roles Traditional Healers Play in Cancer Treatment in Malaysia: Implications for Health Promotion and Education* Asian Pacific Journal of Cancer Prevention, Vol 14, 2013

Figure 56 Miracle Berry (Synsepalum dulcificum)

Fenugreek (Halba) Honey

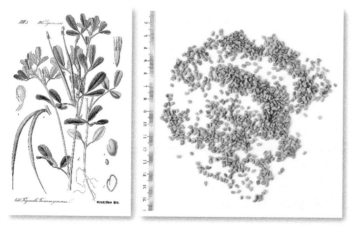

Figure 57 Trigonella foenum-graecum (Fenugreek or Halba)

- Halba (Fenugreek) is helpful for cough problems, sore joints and gout problems.
- Fenugreek (*Trigonella foenum-graecum*) is said to have several health benefits, particularly for women, such as increasing breast milk production, relieving menstrual cramps, and increasing sex drive. It also manages blood sugar levels and body weight.
- Practitioners would infuse the honey of stingless bees with extracts of a nest entrance cerumen with an introitus shape for women's health problems.

---

39 Ansar, A., Lewis, V., McDonald, C., & Liu, C. (2021). Duration of intervals in the care seeking pathway for lung cancer in Bangladesh: A journey from symptoms triggering consultation to receipt of treatment. PLoS One, 16(9), e0257301.

CHAPTER 9

Middle Eastern Remedies and Traditions

Yemen Sidr Honey relation to *Nigella sativa*

- Assorted herbs and spices honey maceration and infusion
- Pollen and propolis capsules and powder for human and poultry feed.
- Premium concoctions like Habatus sauda (Nigella sativa) Honey and Tongkat Ali (Eurycoma longifolia) Honey
- Propolis & Honey Poultices with turpentine oil and flax seed oil for wound healing for humans and pets.

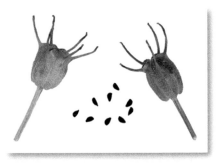

Figure 58 Habatus Sauda Fruit (Black Cumin)

Table 1 Main pollen types of honey samples.

Pollen type	Percentage (%) of pollen			
	Egyptian	Yemeni	Saudi	Kashmir
Sesamum indicum	41	–	12	–
Rhamnus sp.	14	33	5	5
Eucalyptus spp.	1	15	4	11
Trifolium sp.	3	3	12	1
Phoenix dactylifera	20	5	61	31
Nigella sativa	–	20	–	–

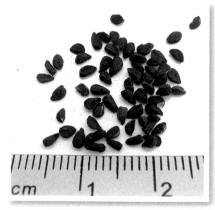 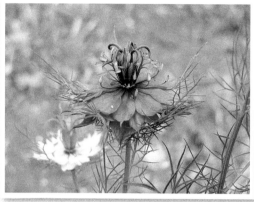 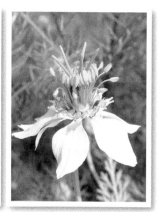

Figure 59 Nigella sativa seeds and flowers can be blue or white.

Nigella Sativa (Black Cumin – Habatus Sauda) Honey - Islamic traditions

- The hadith narrated by 'Aishah R.A., meaning: Truly Habatus sauda', is a cure for all diseases except al-Saam. I asked: What is al-Saam? His Majesty SAW replied: "Death". [Reported by al-Bukhari (5687)]:

- Explanation of scholars: According to Ibn Hajar al-`Asqalani, Habatus sauda' can prevent diseases caused by cold. Among them, when the seeds of Habatus sauda' are crushed and wrapped in a cloth until they emit an aroma, the aroma can help cure people suffering from colds due to cold weather. In addition, Habatus sauda' which has been cooked with vinegar and gargled with it, can relieve toothache.

- In explaining this phrase, Ibn Hajar al-'Asqalani[40] quotes the view of al-Khattabi, who states that "cure for all diseases" is general but has a specific meaning. This is because, according to Imam al-Khattabi, there is not a single plant created by Allah S.W.T. in this world that contains all the benefits for medical purposes.

- Ibn al-Qayyim also mentioned that Habbatus Sauda is useful for treating cold diseases. In addition, it can also treat diseases that are hot and dry due to certain factors. Hot medicine can be used for diseases that are also specifically hot because there has been a lot of evidence that hot medicines can cure diseases that are also hot. For example, hot al-kibriit (sulfur) can treat ringworm or itching.

- Habbatus sauda is from the Arabic term Habat-ul-Sauda and is referred to as Kalonji in South Asia, besides having the English name Black Cumin. Nigella sativa (Habbatus sauda), a plant from the Ranunculaceae family, grows abundantly in several Middle Eastern and Southern Mediterranean countries.

- What hadith say about black cumin seed?

- About the black seed Abu Hurayrah (ra) narrates that the Prophet (pbuh) said: "Hold on (use this seed regularly)! Because it is a remedy (cure) for every disease except death". The above statement indicates that God (Allah) has already created remedies for every disease except death.

- Black cumin is cultivated in the Middle Eastern Mediterranean, Southern Europe, Northern India, Pakistan, Syria, Turkey, Iran, and Saudi Arabia. Nigella sativa seeds and their oil have a

---

40 Irsyad al-Hadith - Pejabat Mufti Wilayah Persekutuan. https://muftiwp.gov.my/en/artikel/irsyad-al-hadith/4702-irsyad-al-hadith-series-517-understanding-the-hadith-habbatussauda-black-cumin-is-a-remedy-to-all-illnesses

long history of folklore usage in Indian and Arabian civilizations as food and medicine (Yarnell and Abascal, 2011)

A well-known physician in the 10ᵗʰ century, Avicenna, wrote a book, "The Canon of Medicine," which recommended using Nigella seeds to enhance the body's energy and also support during recovery from fatigue and dispiritedness.

Ustadza Anisa Taha Arab, a local Muslim Religious Leader based in Cotabato City, said a narration that describes the curative powers of the black seed from Abu Hurairah (ra) said that the Prophet (pbuh) said: "Hold on (use this seed regularly)! Because it is a remedy (cure) for every disease except death".

The medicinal benefits of black seed are mainly due to its main active compound, thymoquinone, which has shown antioxidant, anti-inflammatory, and other therapeutic properties that protect the body from cell damage and chronic diseases. Studies show that black seed is a good source of Calcium, Iron, Zinc, Copper, Thiamine, Niacin, Phosphorous, and Folic Acid. Source[41]

References

- (Musharraf et al. 2018 Prophetic medicine is the cheapest, safest and the best remedy in the prevention and treatment of hypertension (high blood pressure) – a mini-review International *Journal of Molecular Biology Volume 3 Issue 6 eISSN: 2573-2889 https://medcraveonline.com/IJMBOA/ prophetic-medicine-is-the-cheapest-safest-and-the-best-remedy-in-the-prevention-and-treatment-of-hypertension-high-blood-pressure-ndash-a-mini-review.html*)
- Srinivasan, K. 2018 Cumin (Cuminum cyminum) and black cumin (Nigella sativa) seeds: traditional uses, chemical constituents, and nutraceutical effects *Food Quality and Safety, Volume 2, Issue 1, March 2018, Pages 1–16, https://doi.org/10.1093/fqsafe/fyx031*
- Tavakkoli, A. 2017 Review on Clinical Trials of Black Seed (Nigella sativa) and Its Active Constituent, Thymoquinone *J Pharmacopuncture. 2017 Sep; 20(3): 179–193. doi: 10.3831/ KPI.2017.20.021*

Honey and Gastroenterology

Ayyas bin Al Walid has told us Abdul A'la has told us Sa'id from Qatadah from Abu Al Moutawakel from Abu Sa'id that a man came to the Prophet Sallallaahu alaihi wasallam while said, "My brother is suffering from a stomach ache." He said: "Drink honey." Then the man came a second time. Then he kept saying: "Drink honey." Then the man came a third time. He said: "Drink honey." Then he came again saying, "I have done it." So, he said: "Glorious is Allah, and your brother's stomach is a lie, give honey to drink." Then he drank honey and finally recovered. (Bukhari)

Honey has a long history as a treatment for gastrointestinal conditions. Islamic holy scripts[42] dating back to the 8ᵗʰ century show the Prophet Muhammad (pbuh) recommending honey for diarrhoea. Circa 25 AD, Roman physicians prescribed different types of honey to cure diarrhoea and constipation.

41 https://www.nnc.gov.ph/regional-offices/mindanao/autonomous-region-in-muslim-mindanao/6589-black-seed the-seeds-of-healing

42 https://www.frontiersin.org/articles/10.3389/fnut.2022.957932/full

Drinking warm water can soothe the digestive tract and make digestion easier on your stomach. Drinking green tea with raw honey has several potential benefits for healing gastritis. One study showed a significant difference in people with gastritis[43] who drank tea with honey once a week.

Honey: its antibacterial action in treating gastroenteritis (Anon 1985) https://pubmed.ncbi.nlm.nih.gov/12314387/#:~:text=Studies%20have%20confirmed%20that%20honey,the%20duration%20of%20the%20diarrhea.

References:

- El Sohaimy, 2015 *Physicochemical characteristics of honey from different origins* Elsevier B.V. on behalf of Faculty of Agriculture, Ain Shams University.
- Farooq, I., et al., 2022, *Role Of Honey And Nigella Sativa In The Management of COVID-19: HNS-COVID-PK Trial,* CHEST Congress 2022
- Ashraf, S., et al., 2020, *Honey and Nigella sativa against COVID-19 in Pakistan (HNS-COVID-PK): A multi-centre placebo-controlled randomized clinical trial* medRxiv doi: https://doi.org/10.1101/2020.10.30.20217364;
- Korabi M.N.A., et al. 2022, *Comparison between the Efficacy of Nigella sativa-Honey and Clotrimazole on Vulvovaginal Candidiasis: A Randomized Clinical Trial* Hindawi Evidence-Based Complementary and Alternative Medicine Volume 2022, Article ID 1739729, 8 pages https://doi.org/10.1155/2022/1739729
- Najwa, U. A. 2015 *The Miracle of Habatus Sauda According to Islamic and Chemistry Perspective.* Faculty Of Science and Technology UIAM, 2015

---

43   https://www.healthline.com/health/home-remedies-for-gastritis

CHAPTER 10

Derivative Products and By-products.

Papaya Pollination and Honey-Pickled Papaya

Papaya contains all essential vitamins, including vitamins A, C, and minerals like folate, magnesium, copper, etc. Honey is an instant energizer and a bioactive plant compounds and antioxidants powerhouse.

Mash one cup of chopped papaya and mix it with two tablespoons of honey to make a smooth paste. Apply it evenly on your face and neck. Leave it on for 20 minutes and then rinse with cold water. This will help moisturize your skin and bring an instant glow[44].

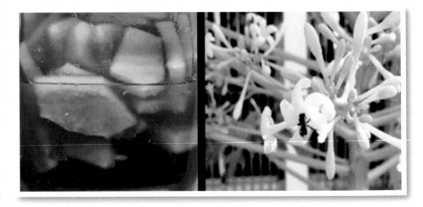

Figure 60 Honey Pickled Papaya and SB on Carica papaya – male flowers

Honey + Coconut water, Sap or Vinegar Beverage

- In the Philippines, Botung for coconut water
- Tuba is newly harvested coconut sap... the daily harvest. Tuba is at least 12 hrs in the aerobic or open air. Bahal for week-old coconut sap
- Bahalina has fermented anaerobically. Vinegar is Suka (Malay= cuka) in Visayan and Tagalog, while Langgaw is an Ilonggo Term for Vinegar.

---

44 https://swirlster.ndtv.com/beauty/3-ways-to-use-papaya-for-glowing-skin-1846496

- Langgaw, in Visayan Terms, is stagnant water. Spicy Vinegar in Ilonggo is Sinamak, Pinakurat in Iligan, while KusisLanggaw is for fermented, months to year-old coconut sap. A.k.a. vinegar. At any of these stages, they may be mixed with honey as a drink
- 2 Tblspn honey +1 Tbspn apple cider or coconut vinegar+ one glass of lukewarm water removes respiratory (COVID) symptoms and even alleviates kidney stones. (Mindanao home-remedy)
- [45][46]Coconut vinegar, derived from fermented coconut sap, is rich in probiotics and acetic acid that can help support a healthy gut. This vinegar has a lighter, sweeter flavour than apple cider vinegar, and you can easily substitute it in recipes that call for ACV in Zamboanga and Bohol.

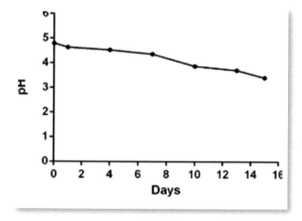

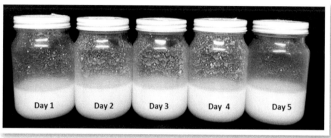

Figure 62 Batch of replicas of the symbiotic drink developed. It was verified that the final formulation was reproducible; batches of the beverage made on five consecutive days, after eight hrs. of incubation, are shown.

Figure 61 pH variation during storage of symbiotic drink.

Rich in probiotics. Natural organic coconut vinegar is rich in probiotics due to the long fermentation process... Rich in polyphenols and nutrients. ... Reduces blood sugar. ... help manage diabetes. ... Suppresses appetite. ... Help you lose weight. ... Aids heart health. ... Helps gut health.

References:

- Prado, E. C., et al., 2015, *Development and evaluation of a fermented coconut water beverage with potential health benefits* Journal of Functional Foods Volume 12, January 2015, Pages 489-497 http://dx.doi.org/10.1016/j.jff.2014.12.020
- Segura-Badilla, O., et al., 2020, *use of coconut water (Cocos nucifera L) for the development of a symbiotic functional drink* Heliyon 6 (2020) e03653 Published by Elsevier Ltd. https://doi.org/10.1016/j.heliyon.2020.e03653
- Gautam, D. et al., 2017, *Nonthermal pasteurization of tender coconut water using a continuous flow coiled U.V. reactor* LWT - Food Science and Technology Volume 83, September 15 2017, Pages 127-131 https://doi.org/10.1016/j.lwt.2017.05.008
- Preetha, P. P., et al., 2013, *Comparative effects of mature coconut water (Cocos nucifera) and glibenclamide on some biochemical parameters in alloxan-induced diabetic rats.* Brazilian Journal of Pharmacognosy 23(3): 481-487, May/Jun. 2013 DOI: 10.1590/S0102-695X2013005000027

---

45 https://doi.org/10.1016/j.heliyon.2020.e03653
    Published by Elsevier Ltd. This is an open access article under the CC BY-NC-ND license (http://creativecommons.org/licenses/bync-nd/4.0/).
46 https://elmarasi.com/en/product/lotus-honey-ginseng-herbal-strength-paste-240-gm

CHAPTER 11

Traditional uses of S.B. honey in Vietnam

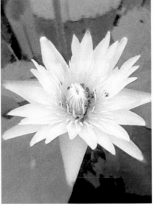

Figure 63 Vietnam Stingless Bees in white water lily (Nymphaea alba) by Trần Quangs

Lotus (*Nelumbo nucifera*), Lily Flower Honey, and Water Lily (*Nymphaea* sp.) Honey

Lotus contains chemicals that decrease swelling, kill cancer cells and bacteria, reduce blood sugar, help break fat, and protect the heart and blood vessels. Chemicals in Lotus also seem to protect the skin, liver, and brain.

Benefits of nutritional Lotus honey past

- Giving the body a large amount of energy to carry out its work and duties
- Getting rid of microbes, viruses, fungi and bacteria and expelling them from the body
- Reducing body fat percentage, combating heart disease, arteriosclerosis and obesity,
- It also lowers the level of cholesterol in the blood
- Protecting the digestive system from infection with many diseases and treating many
- Problems encountered, such as indigestion, constipation, and intestinal infections
- Protecting teeth and protecting them from decay, maintaining healthy gums, and protecting them from infections
- fight against cancer; Because it contains antioxidants.
- Pain relief, and is an effective solution to the problem of insomnia and lack of sleep
- Regulating blood pressure and increasing haemoglobin secretion in the body.

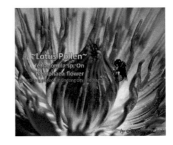

Figure 64 Linh Ling Pagoda in Danang City, Vietnam

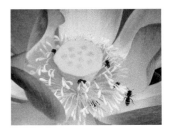

Figure 65 SB on Pink Lotus by Suardi Saide

Lotus Honey Mixed Herbal Paste[47]

Lotus flower honey paste is known as a paste made mainly of natural honey. Adding some other substances to treat some diseases, such as ginseng.

Visiting any major city in Vietnam would put one inevitably with a pond of semiaquatic plants. Lillies and flowering lotus is a common sight because of the religious significance of the flowers. Buddhists revere the lotus flower and even often depict the buddha statue sitting cross-legged on a blooming lotus flower.

As one explores the Vietnamese town market courtyards, there would always be Lotus flowers in bloom in the ponds, and stingless bees are usually foraging in them. Their colourful blooms are alluring and pristine, floating on the glimmering water surface. Some say the bees go to the Lotus to die, and, indeed, one may occasionally find many dead bees on these flowers. However, we have not determined the cause of this phenomenon.

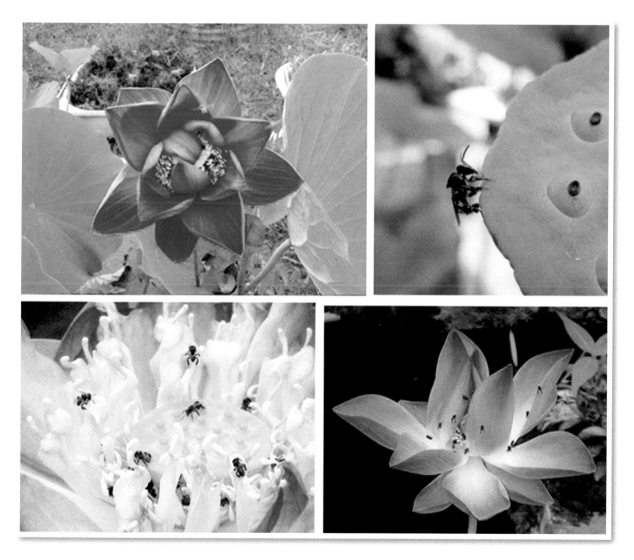

Figure 66 Assorted shapes and colours of the Lotus flower visited by Stingless bees.

47   https://pacificcross.com.vn/honey-benefits/ … Publisher/Author: Pacific Cross Vietnam

(<u>HEALTHCARE</u>)[48] – Honey: Nature's Liquid Gold by Pacific Cross Vietnam

Honey has been considered a folk remedy for thousands of years due to its diversity of medical uses and health benefits. It has so many benefits to our health that people often regard it as "liquid gold" or "food of the gods." Thanks to their versatility, you can eat them raw, processed, or incorporated into other foods as a sweetener. Furthermore, honey has many varieties that can cater to everyone's taste and textural preferences. Some of the most popular ones are manuka honey, clover honey, and multi-flower Honey.

Antioxidant

Honey is rich in antioxidants like flavonoids and polyphenols[49]. Antioxidants are very good for our health since they can fight off inflammation. This property makes honey believed to be able to help us fight off diseases caused by oxidative stress & chronic inflammation and is currently studied for cancer prevention.

Cough relief

Even though over-the-counter medicines are much more effective than honey for cough relief, they are still a great alternative in an emergency. Honey might also be easier to give to smaller children who do not like the taste of cough syrup.

According to Charlotte Smith, MD, a physician at Penn Urgent Care South Philadelphia, Honey is one of the best remedies for a sore throat due to its natural antibacterial properties that allows it to act as a wound healer, immediately offering relief for pain while working to reduce inflammation. Honey can also kill bacteria and help fight off viral infections[50]."

You can take honey directly as it is or dilutes two tablespoons into a glass of warm water to make it easier to drink. There are also herbals like lemon, lime, ginger or mint to add to your glass as a booster or to enhance the taste.

Many of us might have heard about the belief that honey does not expire. It does not get mouldy due to its antibacterial and antifungal properties that discourage bacterial growth. Moreover, honey's high viscosity makes it a less-than-ideal base for microorganisms to live in or reproduce. As a result of these properties, honey is believed to be a powerful aid in fighting infections.

Wound healer

Many studies suggest that honey is effective as a wound healer. On the contrary, some experts believe that honey does not substantially benefit scars or burns. Some researchers have also warned against rubbing honey on open scars, especially for people with diabetes, due to safety risks.

---

48   https://www.thediabetescouncil.com/manuka-honey-and-diabetes/
49   https://asianrecipesathome.com/korean-asian-pear-ginger-tea/
50   https://www.instagram.com/p/CnDY1eqPgqC/

Even though it remains debated in the scientific community, honey has been topically used by indigenous people of Ancient Egypt, Greece, and Rome for wound healing. The sticky consistency of honey keeps the wound moisturized and acts as a protective antimicrobial barrier against infection.

Skin Soothing & Brightening

Honey is becoming an increasingly popular ingredient in skincare formulations. It has humectant properties which can make the skin hydrated and soothed. Even though each product has its properties which differ from one brand to another, skincare that includes honey is usually marketed for people with sensitive skin due to its "skin barrier protecting" properties.

Additionally, propolis harvested from bee farms is included in many skincare products. Due to their high antioxidant content, it is believed to have the ability to help with hyperpigmentation[51] issues — though it is known to be less potent than the popular vitamin C serums. Suppose you suffer from dark spots or would love to see a mild improvement in your complexion brightness, but have sensitive skin that does not tolerate vitamin C serums well, then honey & propolis-based skincare products can be good to consider.

Safety Precautions & Recommendations

Due to the known risk of infant botulism, don't feed honey or products containing honey to children under 12 months.

Honey allergies are rare but possible (approximately <0.001% of the population). Traces of bee pollen and nectar that are accidentally left on honey during the harvesting process can make some people have severe anaphylaxis reactions.

Vanilla Infused Honey

Some benefits of the Vanilla Bean (*Vanilla planifolia*) include Powerful Antioxidants, Antibacterial (Can be used to treat cold sores), Anti Inflammatory, Mental Health boosters, Fever Reducer, and Stabilizing cholesterol.

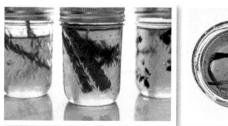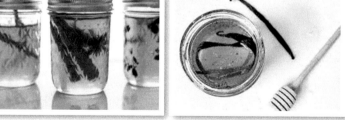

Figure 67 Vanilla beans soaked in Honey

It's a natural preservative with antiseptic qualities that can soothe sore throats, coughs & colds[52]. Vanilla is also beneficial for digestion, stomach problems and inflammation. Tasting notes and tips: Lots of floral notes and the fresh vanilla gives the honey a distinctive 'tang'.

---

51   https://www.fromfieldandflower.co.uk/product/sussex-wildflowers-honey-set-of-two/
52   https://www.linkedin.com/pulse/health-benefits-honey-mixed-aloe-vera-ngoc-anh-bui/

References:

- Thanh, L. N. & Bankova, V., 2017/2018, Searching for bioactive compounds from Vietnamese propolis Vietnam Academy of Science and Technology https://vast.gov.vn/web/vietnam-academy-of-science-and-technology/tin-chi-tiet/-/chi-tiet/searching-for-bioactive-compounds-from-vietnamese-propolis-10316-871.html
- Oanh, VTK, et al., 2021 *New dihydrochromene and xanthone derivatives from Lisotrigona furva propolis* Fitoterapia Volume 149, March 2021, 104821 https://doi.org/10.1016/j.fitote.2020.104821
- Thanh, L. N., et al., 2018, *Isolated Triterpenes from Stingless Bee Lisotrigona furva Propolis in Vietnam* Semantic Scholar - No Paper Link Available
- *Popova, M., Trusheva, B., Bankova, V. (2021). Chemistry and Applications of Propolis. In: Murthy, H.N. (eds) Gums, Resins and Latexes of Plant Origin. Reference Series in Phytochemistry.* Springer, Cham. https://doi.org/10.1007/978-3-030-76523-1_38-1
- Nguyen, T. A. et al., 2017, *Classification and identification of Vietnamese honey using chemometrics based on 1H-NMR data.* Vietnam Journal of Science, Technology and Engineering June 2017 • Vol.59 Number 2
- Georgieva K et al. (2019) *Phytochemical analysis of Vietnamese propolis produced by the stingless bee Lisotrigona cacciae.* PLoS ONE 14(4): e0216074. https://doi.org/10.1371/journal.pone.0216074

12

Traditional uses of SB Honey in Australia

Aloe Vera + Honey Drink

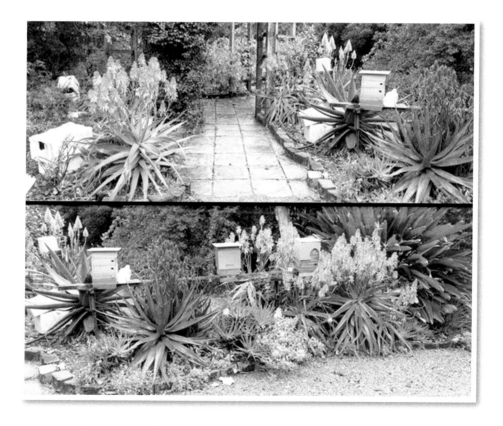

Figure 68 Stingless Bees hives at Bob Lutrell's in Sanford, Queensland.

I had the privilege to visit Bob Lutrell in Sanford, Queensland, and he had an assortment of Aloe Vera of different coloured flowers. Interestingly, he had his hives of stingless bees amidst his plot of the Aloe Vera collection. Though I did not delve into the exclusive taste of Aloe Vera blossom derived honey, I did find some interesting facts on the benefit of drinking aloe vera and honey. Also, aloe vera contains compounds known as polysaccharides which, like raw honey, can reduce the risks and help cure ulcers. Two/ A mixture of honey and aloe vera can also help to boost our overall immunity. This is due to both ingredients containing potent antioxidants that are high in quality[53].

During my stay in Australia, I found some peculiar potential bee-foraging blossoms rarely found in the Indo-Malayan Region. E.g., Orange Blossoms, Banksia, Davidson Sour Plum and Macadamia Nut.

Citrus sinensis – **Orange Blossom**[54] **Honey**

Rich in Vitamin C, it's traditionally used to support the immune system and treat the flu. Like all kinds of honey, it has anti-inflammatory & antiseptic properties. It may be beneficial in soothing and suppressing muscle spasms.

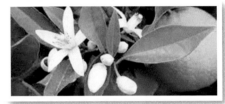

This honey has multiple properties that differentiate it from other kinds of honey. Specifically, it is rich in methyl anthranilate, a unique orange blossom component, giving honey a unique flavour and aroma.

It can be used as a face mask[55] or as a moisturizer for the skin. It also makes a great hair mask to help nourish and condition the hair. The antioxidants and vitamins in the honey can help protect the skin from damage and keep it looking healthy and youthful.

Davidson Sour Plums (*Davidsonia pruriens*) Honey

Davidsonia pruriens, also known as *ooray*, Davidson's plum, or Queensland Davidson's plum, is a medium-sized rainforest tree of northern Queensland, Australia.

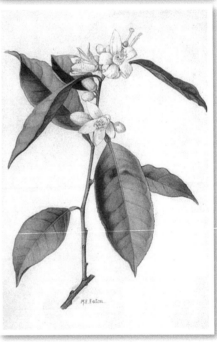

Figure 69 Citrus sinensis - Orange Blossom

A unique dairy-free source of calcium. An antioxidant powerhouse containing high levels of anthocyanin, it is thought to improve cognitive function and protect against certain cancers and heart diseases. A good source of Vitamin E and zinc, two nutrients required for glowing, youthful-looking skin[56]. Davidson Plum is brimming with natural Phyto-compounds, including Tartaric Acid: This natural fruit acid stimulates cell turnover, works as a natural exfoliator and can improve barrier function, helping skin repair and making it look healthy and vibrant.

---

53 https://en.wikipedia.org/wiki/Orange_blossom
54 What you didn't know about honey. (2017, April 13). The Boston Banner, 52(37), 19.
55 https://austsuperfoods.com.au/davidson-plum/
56 https://www.delightedcooking.com/what-is-macadamia-honey.htm

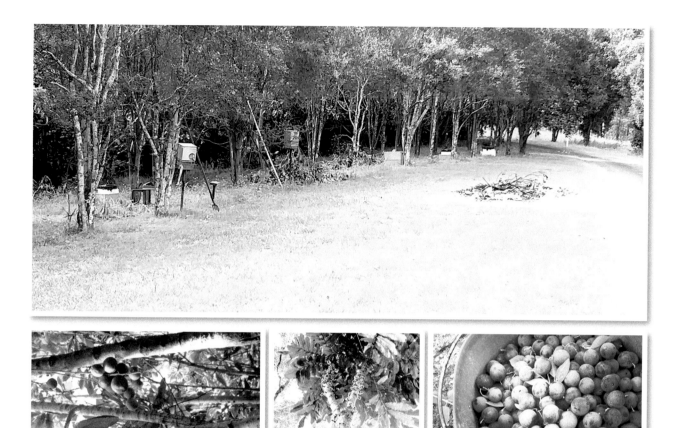

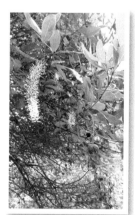

Figure 70 Top: Doug Brownlow @ Camp Mountain, S.E. Queensland with SB hives from Bob Luttrell. Bottom left: Dangling fruits; Middle: Flowers; Right: collected fruits

Macadamia (*Macadamia integrifolia*) Honey

Macadamia honey is a type of honey produced by bees that are placed near macadamia nut tree orchards, where all of their pollination activity is focused on the white flowers that the macadamia nut tree produces. This gives the honey a nutty flavour reminiscent of the macadamia nut itself[57].

Aside from being rich in antioxidants, macadamia honey also contains properties that help treat colds, infections, and flu. The powerful antioxidants present in this

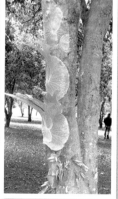

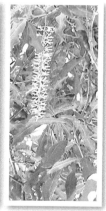

Figure 71 Macadamia flowers at Ken Dorey's Macadamia Farm @ Newrybar

honey effectively fight bacteria that cause the common cold. Besides being rich in antioxidants and natural sweeteners, macadamia honey offers vitamins, minerals, and protein. It can help treat various skin conditions and help in the healing process,

---

57 https://www.australianwoodwork.com.au/pages/banksia

Banksia (*Banksia sp.*) Honey

Banksia Honey is incredibly dark in appearance. It packs a punch with aromas of deep caramel and molasses flavours that will reward the daring. It has a slightly dry mouthfeel and an intense and interesting sweetness. Usually slow to crystallize.

Banksia produce large amounts of nectar and harbour insect larvae that provide[58] food for native wildlife, including birds, insects and small mammals.

The Indigenous people of southwestern Australia would suck on the flower spikes to obtain the nectar. They also soaked the flower spikes in water to make a sweet drink. The Noongar people of southwest Western Australia also used infusions of flower spikes to relieve coughs and sore throats. Source: https://warndu.com/blogs/first-nations-food-guide/ australias-sweet-native-nectar-banksia

Reference:

Irish J, Blair S, Carter DA (2011) *The Antibacterial Activity of Honey Derived from Australian Flora.* PLoS ONE 6(3): e18229. doi:10.1371/ Journal. Pone.0018229

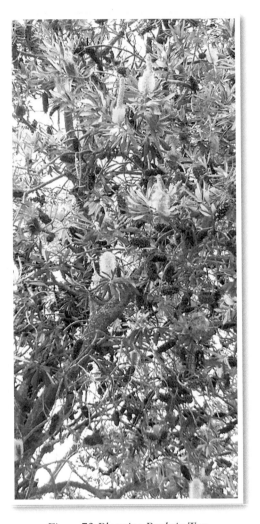

Figure 72 Blooming Banksia Tree at a Gold Coast Beach.

---

58   Editor's Note: Not really. The church needed wax candles, which do not drip. Sustainable was not yet invented, but they certainly were not thinking about food, other than honey.

13

Therapeutic effects of Stingless Bee keeping

Observing stingless bees in their daily activities can be engrossing and have a calming effect on a Beekeeper. It often leaves one pondering for hours, sometimes in awe of nature's intricacies.

Bee pollen is used in the apitherapeutic treatment as it demonstrates a series of actions such as antifungal, antimicrobial, antiviral, anti-inflammatory, immunostimulant, and local analgesic and also facilitates the granulation process of the burn wound healing

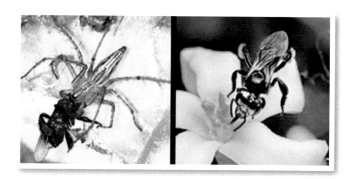

Left: Lynx spider devouring a stingless bee; Right: A Stingless bee foraging nectar on a citrus flower.

Stingless bee honey has been shown to have therapeutic properties, such as antioxidant, antibacterial, and anti-inflammatory properties, and is a natural moisturizer for wound healing applications.

A rare elixir made from the stingless bees in the Land of Happiness.

The Stingless Bees swarm around the thick green vegetation, buzzing in rhythm while storing honey in sack-like wax structures. Their particular honey, Puthka honey in Bhutan, is more commonly known as Meliponine honey (scientific tribe: Meliponini) or stingless-bee honey in other parts of the world.

This nectar is scarce because these bees harvest honey only at 700 to 1500 meters above sea level. A few regions of Bhutan have emerged as the perfect habitat for stingless bees' honey to thrive on, facilitating the production of high-quality Meliponine honey.

Puthka honey's benefits have been widely recognized, making it an interesting item to keep in your pantry or pharmacy.

Its unique taste

Unlike regular honey, the taste of Meliponine honey is uniquely delicious with a sweet-sour essence. It's thinner and more syrup-like. The acidic nature of the honey exudes a tangy taste and has caught the attention of world-famous chefs, such as Rene Redzepi, to implement stingless bees honey as a part of their recipes.

Its creation process

Meliponine bees, commonly known as stingless bees, are generally smaller than regular honeybees. Their small sizes allow them to retrieve more nectars residing deeper in the floral nectaries. The most important portion of the Puthka honey is made of propolis (resinous mixture), formed when the bee salivates on its source of food production (bark, pollen, flowers). After collecting the nectar, the bees store it in their guts. Later, the nectar droplets are ripened through the spinning of the droplets inside their mouths until honey is formed. Each stingless beehive can only produce approximately 700 grams of honey annually, making the Puthka honey rare and precious.

Its collection process

Meliponine bees produce Puthka honey by preserving it in wax structures. When the structures are broken down, the honey pots are squeezed into the form of a chemical-free(organic) product by the farmers of Bhutan.

Extracting Meliponine honey is not easy because the nesting habits of the Meliponine bees are unique and vary. They build their hives in hollow trees and shrubs or even in termite mounds within or under the ground making it difficult for the farmers to reach them. Moreover, the extraction requires experience, as people who do not know about rearing or extracting the honey may destroy entire colonies (hives).

Its scientifically proven health benefits

Thanks to their small size, the Stingless Bees absorb more of the nutritious properties of the plants than other bees. With a higher nutritional value, this honey possesses greater benefits than the ones produced by regular bees. It has been used in traditional medicine for centuries to treat many conditions such as eye, ear, respiratory, digestive, and postpartum conditions, and its usage is becoming more common in modern medicine.

The nutrients available in Meliponine honey are twice as much as the honey produced by regular bees. This honey offers anti-inflammatory, antioxidant, and antibacterial properties. These multi-therapeutic values have been shown to effectively treat tonsillitis and therefore cough and cold but also neutralize eye disorders such as cataracts. The chemo-preventive attribute of Meliponine honey is believed to reduce the spreading of carcinogen cells and is often utilized as an anti-cancer diet in alternative medicine.

With such wondrous benefits, Meliponine honey has become a superfood star in the health and wellness community, where it is often consumed as an immunity booster to avert sickness. Meliponine Honey is only available in a few countries around the globe and in small quantities only.

References:

- Choudhari, M. K. et al. 2013 Anticancer Activity of Indian Stingless Bee Propolis: An In Vitro Study. *Hindawi Publishing Corporation Evidence-Based Complementary and Alternative Medicine Volume 2013, Article ID 928280, 10 pages* http://dx.doi.org/10.1155/2013/928280
- Vongsak1, B. et al. In Vitro Cytotoxity of Thai Stingless Bee Propolis from Chanthaburi Orchard. *Walailak J Sci & Tech 2017; 14(9): 741-747.* http://wjst.wu.ac.th
- Arshad, N. A. et al. 2020 Stingless Bee Honey Reduces Anxiety and Improves Memory of the Metabolic Disease-induced Rats. *Bentham Science Volume 19, Issue 2, 2020 Page: [115 - 126] Pages: 12 DOI: 10.2174/1871527319666200117105133*
- Choudhari, M. K. et al. 2013 Antimicrobial activity of stingless bee (Trigona sp.) propolis used in the folk medicine of Western Maharashtra, India. *Journal of Ethnopharmacology Volume 141, Issue 1, 7 May 2012, Pages 363-367*
- Al-Hatamleh. M. A. I. et al. 2020 Antioxidant-Based Medicinal Properties of Stingless Bee Products: Recent Progress and Future Directions *Biomolecules 2020, 10, 923; doi:10.3390/biom10060923*
- Sajjadi, S. S. et al. 2023 Effect of propolis on mood, quality of life, and metabolic profiles in subjects with metabolic syndrome: a randomized clinical trial *Scientific Reports | (2023) 13:4452 |* https://doi.org/10.1038/s41598-023-31254-y
- Harshad S. K. & Sathiyanarayanan L. 2020 Nutritional and Therapeutic Potential of Propolis: A Review. *Research J. Pharm. and Tech. 2020; 13(7): 3545-3549. doi: 10.5958/0974-360X.2020.00627.7*
- Kustiawan, P.M. et al. Bioactivity of Heterotrigona itama Propolis as Anti-Inflammatory: A Review. *Biointerface Research in Applied Chemistry Volume 13, Issue 4, 2023, 326* https://doi.org/10.33263/BRIAC134.326
- Brodkiewicz Y, et al. 2018 Studies of the biological and therapeutic effects of Argentine stingless Bee Propolis, *Journal of Drug Delivery and Therapeutics. 2018; 8(5):382-392 DOI:* http://dx.doi.org/10.22270/jddt.v8i5.1889
- Kipronol, S. J. et al. 2022 Therapeutic uses of stingless bee honey by traditional medicine practitioners in Baringo County, Kenya. *J. Pharmacognosy Phytother. Vol. 14(3), pp. 27-36, October-December 2022 DOI: 10.5897/JPP2022.0618*

CHAPTER 14

Apiculture to Meliponiculture Historical evolution.

Humans have collected honey for at least 15 thousand years, indicated by cave wall depictions. Bee rearing probably started some 9 thousand years ago, as found in dated pottery used in North Africa. Later, bee domestication for honey and pollination in its crude form must have started during the Pharaohs some 4 to 5 thousand years ago, as seen in hieroglyphs and evident in stored jars of honey found in pyramid tombs of the Pharoahs. (Wikipedia, 2016)

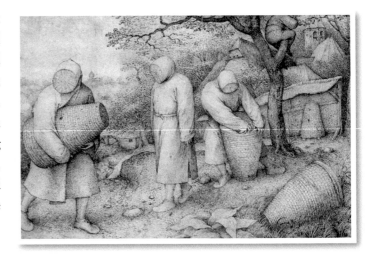

Figure 73 The Beekeepers, 1568, by Pieter Bruegel the Elder

Illustrations in a Medieval health handbook showed some form of Apiculture as far back as the 14th century. It wasn't until the 18th century that European understanding of the colonies and the biology of bees allowed the construction of the moveable comb hive to harvest honey without destroying the entire colony.

However, the Mayans have been rearing stingless bees a few thousand years before. (Roubik 2005). It is from these practices Meliponiculture evolved. In the Maya region, the bee of choice was *Melipona beecheii*, called xuna'an kab or colel-kab ("royal lady") in the Maya language. Bishop Diego de Landa describes the beekeeping practices of domesticated *Melipona beecheii* (the most-used stingless honey bee) and the practices of hunting and collecting honey from wild bees in the forests. (Imre, Young, & Marcus, n.d.)

The Mayans have been at it (Meliponiculture) for the last 2,500 years ago. I refer to a Video titled "Honey for the Maya", a short film by Dr. Stephen Buchmann of the Drylands Institute, Tucson, AZ (https://www.youtube.com/watch?v=d_pjoDxwYS8). It is part of a project he is fundraising for. "I want to finish this project before Dec. 21, 2012". Looking at this dreaded date, I scoured the other videos and one by Elisabeth Theriot. Aptly titled "2012: Why Did the Mayans Predict Armageddon? | Mayan Revelations: Decoding Baqtun" (https://www.youtube.com/watch?v=gK5YJO8wb7w). In this video, she embarks on an epic journey of discovery to dispel the myths about "the December 21st 2012 end of the world" conspiracy theories surrounding Aztec and Mayan Calendars.

Precolumbian Uses of Bees

The domestic use of stingless bees in Mexico dates from pre-Columbian times. This activity reached a particularly impressive level in the Yucatan peninsula, where the Mayan people developed meliponiculture to a level similar to that of management of honey bees during Medieval times in Europe (Quezada-Euán et al., 2001). Accounts of ancient meliponiculture are not abundant in the Americas. Most pre-Columbian evidence comes from Mexico, in particular from the Yucatan Peninsula. Early accounts from Spaniards indicate that outstanding levels of farming and large concentrations of colonies of *Melipona beecheii* ('Xunan kab' in Mayan) were present in the region. An extensive and probably monopolized trade of honey and cerumen with distant territories may have supported the economy and the development of Mayan civilization (Quezada-Euán, 2018). The products of bees, honey and wax[59] were used in Precolumbian Mesoamerica for religious ceremonies, medicinal purposes, as a sweetener, and to make the hallucinogenic honey mead called balche (Hirst, 2016).

Honey Hunting & Beekeeping

Early humans relied on hunting wild animals and gathering vegetables and fruits, and while their hunter-gatherer lifestyle, they would have come across honey in bees' nests high in the trees. Bees provided our ancestors with perhaps their first condiment—honey. This complex concoction was alluring, and its desire drove men to work in groups to capture the golden prize. Their stories are documented in art, and cave drawings from the late Stone Age show a deeply rooted association between humans and bees. Artworks dating to thirteen thousand years depict amazing feats, with men scaling impossibly tall trees, risking falls and stings, and passing the sweet comb down to helpers below. At first, this bravery was the only way of harvesting honey, and it was several thousand years before the refined practice of beekeeping was developed.

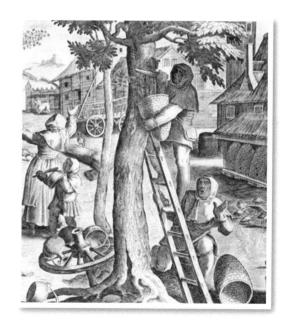

Figure 74 Beekeepers, from "Venationes, Ferrum, Avium, Piscium" (Of Hunting: Wild Beasts, Birds, Fish), engraved by Jan Collaert (1566–1628).

---

59   Editor's Note: You kind of forget the later arrival of Africanized honeybee form Africa, which arrived in Panama in 1984 and in Central America in 1985, where there were NEVER honey bees of any kind living in the wild (by honey bees here, I mean genus Apis).

Ancient Egypt

Some three thousand years old, the earliest known human-constructed beehive was discovered in Israel, but the Ancient Egyptians were the first known beekeepers. Evidence from cave drawings in Egypt reveals a long history of beekeeping, dating to at least 2400 BCE and thought to go back as far as 5000 BCE. The Egyptians first relied on wild bee nests, but their beekeeping practices advanced. Not only did they construct beehives in the form of woven baskets covered in clay, which stayed perma- gently

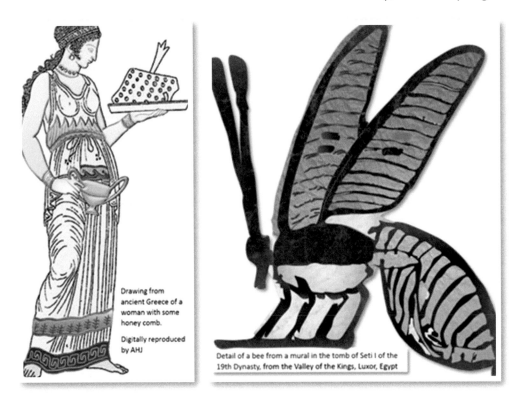

Drawing from ancient Greece of a woman with some honey comb.

Digitally reproduced by AHJ

Detail of a bee from a mural in the tomb of Seti I of the 19th Dynasty, from the Valley of the Kings, Luxor, Egypt

Figure 75 Drawing from ancient Greece of a woman with some honeycomb.

They also used migratory hives in one location, which floated down the River Nile on rafts, producing unique honey blends as the bees visited the ever-changing riverside flowers. Egyptians favoured the honey bees, the best local honey producers.

Environment: Through artificial selection, they gave evolution a helping hand to produce a new subspecies, the Egyptian honey bee (*Apis mellifera lamarckii*). Some beekeepers were likely a lower class of workers forced to work with these aggressive bees and return glorious honey to their superiors and eventually to the pharaohs and the gods. Official guards accompanied other honey harvesters to explore deep into the sur- rounding land, searching for wild hives, low-lying bushes and tall trees. (Wilson-Rich et al. 2014)

Mesoamerica

The people of Mesoamerica (Mexico, Belize, Guatemala, El Salvador, Costa Rica, Honduras, and Nicaragua) kept stingless bees for two thousand years before Europeans brought the western honey bee to their shores. There are likely at least 250 stingless bee species in Brazil and at least 4,000 bee species native to North America alone, but the western honey bee is not native to the Americas[60]. The practice of beekeeping with honey bees was introduced to the New World by Europeans in the seventeenth century as a means of sustainable food production. Some honey bee colonies escaped their beekeepers' management and flew into the woods in this unexplored new land. Native Americans named these feral honey bees "white man's flies" as their arrival announced the advance of the settlers and gave warning of the in- evitable conflict over land that lay ahead. (Wilson-Rich et al. 2014)

Considerations

The ancient Egyptians offered honey to their deities as a sacrifice (36). They also used honey for embalming the dead. Honey was utilized for its antibacterial properties that helped heal infected wounds. Moreover, honey was used as a topical ointment[61].

The type of crops and season, too, had a direct relation to the moisture content of the resultant harvested honey. We had difficulty quantifying the relation because the bees are polylectic in that they forage whichever source was available then.

However, we can predict an estimated volume of regularly scheduled harvesting in monoculture farms or forests with a dominant vegetation type. In such instances, we can ascertain the peculiar benefits of those types of honey. Another instance is where the bee is affixed to a certain type of vegetation and is even dependent on such vegetation. A good example is the species that depend on Dipterocarp resin; in that way, we will be sure that the honey will have resinous micro propolis. This will influence the taste, aroma and, to a certain extent, the colour.

We may conduct more studies to determine a variety of types of vegetation or the biological family of a tree. Hence, we explore as many crops and types of honey as possible to see if we may determine a more direct relation of crop blossom to honey taste, colour and aroma profile.

Propolis

Propolis is a resin-like material made by bees from the buds of poplar and cone-bearing trees. Bees use it to build hives, and it may contain beehive by-products.

Propolis seems to help fight against bacteria, viruses, and fungi. It might also have anti-inflammatory effects and help the skin heal. Propolis is rarely available in its pure form. It's usually obtained from beehives.

People commonly use propolis for diabetes, cold sores, swelling and sores inside the mouth. It's also used for burns, canker sores, genital herpes, and many other conditions, but no good scientific evidence supports these uses. There is also no good evidence to support using propolis for COVID-19.

---

60 https://en.wikipedia.org/wiki/History_of_wound_care
61

Uses & Effectiveness

<u>Possibly Effective for</u>

Diabetes. Taking propolis by mouth seems to improve blood sugar control by a small amount in people with diabetes. But it doesn't seem to affect insulin levels or improve insulin resistance.

Cold sores (Herpes labialis). Applying an ointment or cream containing 0.5% to 3% propolis five times daily might help cold sores to heal faster and reduce pain.

Swelling (inflammation) and sores inside the mouth (oral mucositis). Taking propolis by mouth or rinsing the mouth with a propolis mouth rinse heals sores caused by cancer drugs.

There is interest in using propolis for many other purposes, but there isn't enough reliable information to say whether it might be helpful.

Side Effects

When taken by mouth: Propolis is possibly safe when used appropriately. It can cause allergic reactions, especially in people allergic to other bee products. Lozenges containing propolis can cause irritation and mouth ulcers.

When applied to the skin: Propolis is possibly safe when used appropriately. It can cause allergic reactions, especially in people allergic to other bee products.

Pregnancy: There isn't enough reliable information to know if propolis is safe when pregnant. Stay on the safe side and avoid use.

Breastfeeding: Propolis is possibly safe when taken by mouth while breastfeeding. Doses of 300 mg daily for up to 10 months have been used safely. Stay on the safe side and avoid higher doses when breastfeeding.

Bleeding conditions: A certain chemical in propolis might slow blood clotting. Taking propolis might increase the risk of bleeding in people with bleeding disorders.

Allergies: Some propolis products might be contaminated with bee by-products. Use propolis with caution if you are allergic to bee by-products.

Surgery: A certain chemical in propolis might slow blood clotting. Stop taking propolis two weeks before surgery. Taking propolis might increase the risk of bleeding during and after surgery.

Interactions

<u>Moderate Interaction</u>

Be cautious with this combination

Medications that slow blood clotting (Anticoagulant / Antiplatelet drugs) interact with PROPOLIS

Propolis might slow blood clotting. Taking propolis and medications that slow blood clotting might increase the risk of bruising and bleeding.

Medications changed by the liver (Cytochrome P450 1A2 (CYP1A2) substrates) interacts with PROPOLIS

Some medications are changed and broken down by the liver. Propolis might change how quickly the liver breaks down these medications. The breaking down could change the effects and side effects of these medications.

Warfarin (Coumadin) interacts with PROPOLIS

Warfarin is used to slow blood clotting. This disease might increase the risk of clotting. Propolis might decrease the effects of warfarin.

<u>Dosing</u>

Adults have most often used Propolis in doses of 400-500 mg by mouth daily for up to 13 months. It's also used in many products, including creams, ointments, gels, and mouth rinses. Speak with a healthcare provider to determine the best product and dose for a specific condition. Source: <u>https://www.webmd.com/vitamins/ai/ingredientmono-390/propolis</u>.

Inferences

- Ancient practices, be it a placebo effect or not, must be tried out, tested and compared with control.
- Muslim scholars do not question but reflect on Islamic healing concepts, principles and theology. Either believe, surrender with acceptance or not, although tests and research to further understand are not discouraged.
- Myths and traditional unproven concoctions have to be taken with "a pinch of salt", especially in palliative situations. Otherwise, discard it as an "old wives' tale".
- Many studies and research are needed to understand further "indigenous knowledge". Many properties of the host plant are presumed to be transferred to the nectar and subsequently to the honey produced.

References for the History Section

1. Hirst, K. K. (May 2016). Ancient Maya Beekeeping: Stingless Bee *Melipona beecheii (Ancient Domestication of the American Stingless Bee)*. Retrieved from About Education: http://archaeology.about.com/od/Domesticated-Animals/fl/Ancient-Maya-Beekeeping-The-Stingless-Bee-Melipona-beecheii.htm
2. Imre, D. M., Young, L., & Marcus, J. (n.d.). Ancient Maya Beekeeping (ca. 1000-1520 CE). The *University of Michigan Undergraduate Research Journal*.

3. Roubik, D. W. (June 16 2005). Mayan Stingless Bee Keeping: Going, Going, Gone? *Smithsonian Tropical Research Institute.* Retrieved from https://www.sciencedaily.com/releases/2005/06/050615062105.htm

4. Wikipedia. (September 28 2016). *Beekeeping.* Retrieved from Wikipedia: https://en.wikipedia.org/wiki/Beekeeping

5. Wilson-Rich, N., Allin, K., Carreck, N., Quigley, A., The Bee a Natural History, *Ivy Press* 2014

6. G. Quezada-Euán, J.J. The Past, Present, and Future of Meliponiculture in Mexico; Stingless Bees of Mexico pp 243-269, *Springer Link.* (First Online: 04 August 2018)

7. G. Quezada-Euán, J.J., et al., Meliponiculture in Mexico: problems and perspective for development; Bee World 82(4): 160–167 (2001), *IBRA*

LIST OF FIGURES

INDEX

ABOUT THE AUTHOR

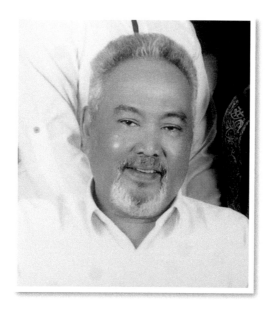

Abu Hassan bin Abdul Jalil (Born 1955)

Began Bee culture career as an Apiary Landscaper as early as 1983, dabbled in Meliponary Landscaping since 2010, and engaged fully in Meliponiculture as of 2011. Actively involved in Indo-Malayan Meliponine Conservation since 2012 by evolving the new study of Beescape for Meliponines.

Beescape and Meliponine Repository Consultant at the Malaysian Genome and Vaccine Institute (MGVI) – 2014 to present.
Principal at Akademi Kelulut Malaysia – 2014 to present.
Member of National Bee Council, MOA, Malaysia – 2022 to present

Author/Co-author on the related subject:
Beescape for Meliponines – Partridge Publishing Singapore 2014
Handbook of Meliponiculture Vol.1 & 2 - AKM 2017
World Meliponine Etymology of Taxonomic Nomenclature – IBRA 2021
Malaysian Meliponiculture & Beyond – IBRA 2021
Geometry & Colours of Meliponine Brood Cells - IBRA 2022
Indonesian Meliponiculture & Beyond - IBRA 2022
Meliponiculture & Beyond in The Philippines - IBRA 2023

Printed in the United States
by Baker & Taylor Publisher Services